What they
never tell you

What they never tell you

Secrets and strategies for surviving the first 6 months of motherhood

Kay Stammers

Published 1997 by Mandarin
a part of Reed Books Australia
35 Cotham Road, Kew, Victoria 3101
a division of Reed International Books Australia Pty Ltd

Copyright © text and photographs, Kay Stammers, 1997

All rights reserved. Without limiting the rights under copyright above, no part of this publication may be reproduced, stored in or introduced into a retrieval system, or transmitted in any form or by any means (electronic, mechanical, photocopying, recording or otherwise), without the prior written permission of both the copyright owner and the publisher.

Designed by David Rosemeyer
Typeset in Australia by Emtype Desktop Publishing Services
Printed and bound by Australian Print Group

National Library of Australia
cataloguing-in-publication data:
  What they never tell you: secrets and strategies for surviving the first six months of motherhood
  Includes index
  ISBN 1 86330 567 X
  1. Infants – Care. 2. Infants – Health and hygiene. 3. Parenthood. I. Title.

649.122

The opinions contained within this book are those of the author. Neither the author nor the publisher accepts any liability for difficulties of any kind arising as a result of any opinion, advice, recommendation or information expressly or implicitly published in or in relation to this publication.
   The author and the publisher of this book are not medically trained and are not licensed to give medical advice. Always consult your doctor if you are uncertain whether your baby's health and development are within the normal parameters.

Contents

ACKNOWLEDGEMENTS vii
INTRODUCTION 1
HOW TO READ THIS BOOK 5
SHOPPING TIPS FOR THE FIRST 6 MONTHS 7

CHAPTER 1	Birth to 1 week	24
CHAPTER 2	1 week old	60
CHAPTER 3	2 weeks old	92
CHAPTER 4	3 weeks old	108
CHAPTER 5	1 month old (4–7 weeks)	126
CHAPTER 6	2 months old (8–11 weeks)	152
CHAPTER 7	3 months old (12–16 weeks)	176
CHAPTER 8	4 months old (17–21 weeks)	192
CHAPTER 9	5 months old (22–25 weeks)	210
CHAPTER 10	6 months and beyond	234

HELP LINES 238
INDEX 243

This book is dedicated to our beautiful son, Rupert, who provided the inspiration, much of the source material, and changed our lives forever. And to his paternal grandmother, Joan, who shines in him, but who sadly died before they could meet.

Acknowledgements

Ideally, parenthood is a partnership, and I am fortunate in having a wonderful, supportive partner to share my voyage of discovery. Tristan was passionately interested in our baby's development, and so made an excellent sounding board and contributor. His insights are reflected in 'A father's view' at the end of each chapter.

Of course, the book had to be believed in to be published and for this I thank my literary agent Margaret Connolly, publisher Jennifer Byrne, publisher's assistant Juanita Crowley, and editor Kirsten Alexander — all, coincidentally, new mothers. Special thanks to Jennifer and Kirsten for their expertise, empathy and undying faith in the book.

After the first draft was completed, I began a thorough research and testing period. I sat in on many postnatal classes, chatted with the mothers, and attended their coffee gatherings. My thanks to those mums for their time and their tips. I'm indebted to the Cremorne Early Childhood Centre for happily playing host to me on these occasions. Thanks, also, to the hospitals which allowed me to sit in on their parents' groups: St Margaret's, the Mater, and the Royal North Shore in Sydney.

As each subsequent draft of the book materialised, I bounced it off new parents. Considering how busy and stressful it is to be a new parent, I'm doubly grateful to all those who generously took the time to read the manuscript and offer valuable feedback: Beverley Stammers, Tanya and David Hain, Anna Booth and Malcolm Scott, Margaret Connolly, Juanita Crowley, Carol Searle, Helen Temple, Joanne Elvey, Beverley Batey, Sue and Roland Everingham, Anne and Craig Buller, Karen Clawson, Trish Cushmore, Margaret Gerard, Natalie Bowra, Sharon Atherton, Jenny Ann Dawes and Teresa Lincoln.

Certain sections needed checking by the relevant experts, and for that I'm indebted to Tresillian Family Care Centres, Karitane, the Nursing Mothers' Association of Australia, the National SIDS Council of Australia, the late Dr Reuben Dubois (formerly Director of Paediatrics, Westmead Hospital), Sally Hanna (Nursing Unit Manager, St Margaret's Hospital), Sue Crisp (lactation consultant), Mary Lantry (NSW Lactation College), Rhonda Reilly (Clockwork Childcare Group), Sandra Bennett (Small Change, Neutral Bay) and the staff of Baby Savings at Willoughby.

I'm immensely grateful to the health professionals who read the manuscript and added comments borne of experience and expertise: Pam Buddle (formerly with Tresillian, now a social worker in private practice), Anne Scollen (lactation advisor, North Shore and Beyond), Angela Martin (midwife and new mother), Aileen Malloy (Acting Manager, Tresillian Family Care Centre, Willoughby) and Kath Youngman (Clinical Nurse Specialist and Co-ordinator, Dalwood Family Care Centre).

Special thanks to Susan Prescott (Clinical Nurse Specialist, Cremorne Early Childhood Health Centre) and Lindy Danvers (Nursing Unit Manager, Chatswood Child and Family Health Service), who both put in generous amounts of time.

My thanks to you all for helping to provide a true picture of the first six months.

Introduction

What They Never Tell You is a collection of the best practical advice I have found to help you through that most awesome stage of a baby's upbringing — from birth to 6 months. It's arranged clearly and chronologically, so that you can easily find and scan the section relating to you and your baby's needs at any particular week or month. It's not meant to cover every conceivable topic, but to present a practical overview, fill in the gaps, and give a sensible, down-to-earth look at your options. It's a book I would have liked to have had, to help me through what I found was a frustrating and gruelling — albeit rewarding and exhilarating — period of motherhood.

Although it's aimed primarily at those having their first baby, many second-time parents will also benefit. After all, it's amazing how rapidly we forget most of the details of bringing up baby. And the help available now wasn't always there the first time around. For example, some of the convenient devices which mothers today take for granted — like Snappy nappy clips to fasten nappies, and steam sterilisers for bottles — weren't on the market in the early nineties.

The information is based on my experience as a first-time mother, and that of many other mothers I've talked to, as well as advice gleaned from the experts — child health nurses in particular. The expression

WHAT THEY NEVER TELL YOU

'what they never tell you' certainly doesn't refer to the many wonderful carers who staff child health and family care services. They can be a fund of practical information. But, unfortunately, many first-time mothers don't seek help soon enough, or perhaps don't even realise that they need help at all. Some are too afraid to ask, or fear they will be taking up too much of the carer's time.

Many books on the market offer valuable advice, but who's got time to wade through them? Often they're sectioned into broad issues such as sleeping or feeding during the first 12 months, when all you want to know is what to do this month. Besides, the long-time favourites, if not recently updated, can be way behind the times.

Often the most useful advice is the sort you'd never expect to find in a book: the tips you pick up from another new mum over a cup of coffee, like bathing your newborn in the bathroom basin, or using a laundry basket as a cosy, supportive playpen for your 3-month-old. Ingenious solutions, often born out of the desperation only a new mother knows. I hope to pass many of these tips on to you. But remember, everyone's experience is different, depending on the baby and your situation. My husband, Tristan, and I were both older parents with many years in the workforce behind us before our baby, Rupert, came along. We were used to positions of responsibility, used to being in control of our careers and our lives, so the demands of a newborn may have hit us harder than it would younger parents without such deeply ingrained routines.

As a television reporter, I chose to continue a light workload when Rupert was 6 weeks old. It was only part-time work, but it brought with it burdens such as expressing milk and seeking out childcare. In addition, I was keeping a diary and editing my first book, written during my pregnancy. As we were living in a two-bedroom apartment, our office had to double as a nursery when the baby was 3 months! (We waited until Rupert was 6 months before moving to a house.) We had no network of family nearby, and our friends were all professional couples either with no children or children who were teenagers or young adults. So we lacked the support structure that many new parents have and also lacked any first-hand knowledge of babies. We had to go it alone. You, on the other hand, might be wondering what the big fuss is about!

INTRODUCTION

Lost in the grim determination of learning how to cope, it took me until the 2-month mark to realise that I could lighten up a little, and start appreciating the joys of having a new baby. And, of course, once the mother relaxes and has some fun with her baby, the benefits multiply. It's a shame no-one tells us how important it is to find a way off that treadmill, to let go of the stress and savour all the fascinating stages of your child's growth. Bringing up baby is a serious business, but many of us — particularly professional mums, I suspect — take it far *too* seriously!

I don't want to distort the wonderful experience of motherhood, but because this book is about problem solving, it naturally focuses on many of the more challenging aspects of caring for a new baby. If these seem to outweigh the positives, rest assured that, in our minds, nothing — nothing! — beats the absolute joy of having your first child.

How to read this book

In my opinion, the first 4 weeks is when you are most in need of guidance. For this reason, I have sectioned the book week by week until the 4-week (1-month) mark, and then month by month until 6 months. Within the monthly sections, there are chronological diary entries relating to each specific week.

When talking about the age of the baby, I prefer the tags we use in everyday conversation, that is, '1 week old', rather than 'the second week' (or week 2), which confuses the issue. Some books, for example, refer to 'the third month', meaning the passage of time between when baby turns 2 months and when he turns 3 months. It is much clearer to just say '2 months old', which is what he is!

Because there is more information to pack into the first 4 weeks, you'll find these chapters quite long, compared with chapters in the last half of the book. Rather than attempt to balance the length of the chapters, I have let them 'write themselves', according to what is relevant for that particular stage.

The book is meant to be read in stages, so you may find there is some repetition. This is because parents picking up the book at 3 months cannot necessarily expect to have remembered what they read at the 2-week stage. In any case, techniques (for example, for settling) will be slightly different at different ages. There will also be more detailed information added about certain subjects as the book progresses. I have allowed for the fact that in the early stages parents have a lot to digest and in some areas knowledge needs to be built up gradually.

When reading the 'Milestones' sections at the beginning of each chapter, bear in mind that babies develop at their own individual pace. Your baby may do some things earlier, or later, than the guide given. The span of 'average' can be very broad (for example, the average age for walking is anything from 12 to 18 months!). There are many factors which can influence a baby's development, such as hereditary characteristics or how much love, time and attention he gets. So don't panic (or gloat) if your baby isn't going exactly by the book, or doing what a friend's baby is doing this week. Chances are he's coming along just fine, and shouldn't be rushed to achieve his goals. If in doubt, ask your child health nurse. (I use the term 'child health nurse' to refer to qualified carers in this area and 'child health centre' to refer to your local child clinic. Titles vary from state to state.)

At the end of each chapter, my husband, Tristan, has shared his feelings relating to that stage. His comments, born out of intimate and enthusiastic participation in the caring process, are directed particularly at other new fathers.

Please note that the names of health professionals referred to in this book are not necessarily their real names.

Finally, I have used 'he' throughout, with apologies to those who have 'shes'. I feel that alternating sexes each chapter is a cumbersome way of overcoming the gender problem, so I've chosen to be consistent with the authentic diary extracts, which refer to my own baby boy.

Shopping tips for the first 6 months

It's not only more fun to do much of the baby shopping beforehand, it's essential. There's just not the time or opportunity during the weeks following delivery to skip out to the store every time you need to pick up a few extras — unless you're very organised or have lots of help. Even then, you'll be glad if you have everything on hand for the first few months.

However, don't, in your excitement, buy too many clothes. You could well find they're for the wrong size, sex or season or you may be given lots of outfits as gifts. And don't go overboard with expensive clothes for 'best'. Babies grow so quickly that you'll be lucky to get more than one wear out of some outfits. And they make such a mess that you'll think twice about dressing them in something which can't be thrown in the washing machine or which needs to be ironed. Easy to wash and dry, non-iron clothing is what you'll appreciate.

Peruse local street stalls, school fetes and country craft markets — they're often a great source of handmade treasures like bibs, blankets and bunny rugs. Some people browse through second-hand shops in the wealthier suburbs to find great outfits at low prices. Of course, you can pick up bargains at garage sales, but you have to be careful they're not shoddy, faulty or superseded.

Many new mothers buy heaps of things, only to find out later that a different model or type would have been more efficient or practical.

If only they'd told me I'd have bought

Large sizes

Choose items which err on the large, rather than the small, side. We found that our baby, 4 kilograms (9 pounds) at birth, couldn't fit into some of the 000 jumpsuits we'd bought. In fact, he was soon into the 3-month versions. Not everyone has a big baby, but it doesn't hurt to have clothing a bit roomy at first — at least he'll get a couple of months' wear out of them.

If, on the other hand, you have a very wee baby, you can always pick up a few 000s at the hospital shop before you leave.

Double terry-towelling bibs

You'll need lots and lots of them. Look for big bibs with small necks for better coverage. Choose those with elastic around the neck, or velcro fasteners, which are easy to whip on and off. Bibs which tie at the neck are too fiddly, especially when you're in a hurry and the baby's wriggling. They invariably form knots and baby's hair can get caught up in the ties. Don't buy the plastic-backed ones — they're too stiff, not as absorbent, and won't go in the tumble dryer.

Especially if you have a posseting baby (you'll soon find out), make sure the bib is wide enough to cover the shoulders and extends around the back of the neck, to catch those unexpected vomits. The fancy little cotton or lace numbers are useless. I don't care where you're going — who needs a decorative, non-absorbent bib?

Jumpsuits

These are all-in-one outfits, which cover baby from neck to toe. Choose those with zips or press-studs not only down the front but also along the inside leg if possible — this makes nappy changing much easier. Jumpsuits are especially good for winter babies. Try to resist those cute French and Italian numbers (even if you can afford them!) which have a buttoned flap at the back and no opening at the front. These are a real hassle each time you change a nappy, although their one advantage is that when you do eventually get them unbuttoned (after doubling baby over uncomfortably on the changing table) they are well clear of his dirty bottom, and the soiled nappy.

Nighties
Buy at least three or four. They make changing nappies during the night a whole lot easier than undoing press-studs or buttons and pulling both little legs out, when you, and the baby, are half asleep.

Separates
T-shirts, sweatshirts and pants are very useful when baby is older, as you can re-use one half of the outfit if the other gets dirty, and they're easy to get on and off. But if you use them between birth and 6 months baby is likely to end up with a bare tummy.

Singlets
Choose those which stretch easily over the head and arms. They're on and off frequently, and tend to cause the baby a great deal of annoyance in the process if they are narrow or tight. (He'll also grow out of them very quickly.) I used a cotton and polyester mix all year round, although you can buy woollen ones for winter if you prefer. My favourites were shaped more like a sleeveless T-shirt with scooped neck, and were very soft, stretchy and comfortable. You can also get them with long sleeves, which some mothers prefer at night.

Socks
Buy at least six pairs of cotton ones, which come in great colours or stripes. I prefer these to knitted or crocheted bootees. As well as looking cute, they stay on and fit snugly under jumpsuits with feet if it's cold. Deflating for grandmothers and aunties, I know, but in my opinion bootees really are a nuisance! Apart from falling off, they're fiddly to do up, and the laces get lost in the washing machine. Ask grandma to knit a little cap or baby blanket instead.

Nappies
Cloth or disposables is obviously a personal choice. Cloth are environmentally better and cheaper. Disposables are far less work, last longer and keep baby drier but, of course, there is the problem of disposing of them. (Be prepared for a kitchen bin stuffed with used disposables which, depending on where you live, may cause your weekly garbage output to exceed the local council quota.) If you

decide on cloth, you'll still appreciate having some disposables in the cupboard for going out, or going away. Some people also prefer them for overnight use, so they don't have to change baby during night feeds. You may choose to use disposables for the first few weeks, until you find your feet.

If you're using cloth, with 8 or more nappies per day you'll need to buy at least 20 to start off with (more if you don't have a clothes dryer). Remember to ask a friend or relative to give you a month's nappy wash service as a gift. It's hard enough keeping up the supply of clean clothes and bunny rugs, let alone adding 60 to 70 dirty nappies a week to your household chores! You can also use this as a trial period, to see if cloth nappies suit you.

Be aware that there are two types of cloth nappies: flannel and towelling. Again, it's a personal choice — flannel is softer, towelling is more absorbent.

You can also buy fitted cloth nappies with velcro fasteners, but they're usually expensive and take much longer to dry.

Nappy liners
You have the choice of disposable or cloth. Some varieties are more effective than others at drawing away wetness from the baby's skin and therefore helping to prevent nappy rash; others make disposing of the contents easier. It's best to try several types and decide which suits you, and baby, best.

Pilchers
You'll need lots (well, at least 7 pairs) if you're using cloth nappies. Pilchers are the waterproof panties which (usually) stop the flood from soaking the jumpsuit. I found that every time the nappy got really wet or dirty, so did the pilchers, which meant frequent changing and washing. Straight-out plastic pants are no-go (hot and humid, ideal for fostering nappy rash).

It's best to get pilchers with velcro fastenings (so you can adjust them as baby gets plumper) or press-studs, rather than the panty type you have to drag on. You can buy basic white, or invest in the more expensive coloured and patterned variety, which often come in boxes (great for baby gifts!). Some mothers with babies prone to nappy rash swear by the fluffy, more absorbent pilchers. (You can also put these in the dryer. Velcro fasteners tend to curl.)

Snappy nappy fasteners
These are great if you're using towelling nappies. I never did get the hang of safety pins, let alone the art of folding. The baby's nappy would be down around his knees in minutes. But now there's a wonderful device that revolutionises cloth nappy use: plastic tension clips, which snap onto towelling and are simply pulled to adjust the nappy to the firmness you desire. What magic! Buy coloured ones so they're easier to find amongst the pile of nappies and pilchers at change time. But beware, they can cause scratches if they come undone, which is why some hospitals don't recommend them. Some hospitals teach a method of nappy folding which allows you to get away without using any pins or fasteners at all for the first few weeks, when baby is less mobile.

Nappy bucket
Buy two if you plan to use cloth nappies: one for the baby's room (to dump the soiled nappies in after changing), and one for the laundry (full of NapiSan, with the lid on for safety reasons). When you've emptied the laundry bucket into the washing machine, you can swap buckets.

Change table
Some mothers try to get by without them, but it's really hard on your back. If you haven't the space or money for a heavy wooden one with all the drawers, shelves and trimmings, a simple plastic and tubular steel fold-up number is just as effective. As well as for changing, they're handy to use for dressing and baby massage. A cheap alternative is a thin piece of foam which you can cover in vinyl or plastic and place on your dressing table.

Bunny rugs
You'll want at least 6 or 7 cotton rugs to wrap baby in. (They dirty them at a rapid rate, either bringing up milk or wetting them through their nappies.) Bunny rugs are really cheap at department stores, although it's nice to shop around and find a couple with bright

interesting patterns, rather than the standard pastels. They can vary slightly in size — buy larger, rather than smaller, ones. You'll be using them continually to swaddle and cover baby in the bassinet, pram, and around the house. They're also good to put on the floor, for baby to lie on. If you want to make your own, buy a fine flannelette sheet and cut it into 1-metre squares. In warmer weather, many mothers like to use muslin wraps for swaddling. Or you can use cot sheets, folded in half — you'll need to buy these at some stage anyway.

Cellular cotton blankets
These are the open-weave type, used in most hospitals. They're light, easy to clean, help avoid overheating the baby, and you can use more for extra warmth.

Cradle or bassinet
Many can be rocked or jiggled lengthways as well as from side to side. This seems to be the most soothing movement to get baby to sleep. A bassinet on wheels is handy, as it can be moved from room to room when necessary. If it separates from its stand, it becomes a portable bassinet, useful for sleeping baby when you go to a friend's place for dinner. I prefer cradles made of cane, with handles. As well as looking good and being light to rock (you can do it with one hand from your bed!), they can be easily carried to the car.

A bassinet is not essential — you can put baby straight into a cot if you prefer, although most people switch to a cot at around 2 to 3 months.

Dimmer or night light
Choose a small plug light, or a stand-alone model. It is important for your bedroom, or nursery (wherever you feed during the night), to avoid having to switch on the main light. It'll also come in handy when your baby is a toddler and won't go to sleep in total darkness.

Woollen underblanket or proof mat
Choose one which is water repellent rather than plastic. If you buy 2 bassinet-sized proof mats — which you need anyway, if one is in the wash — you can later use them side by side in the cot. Or try a

lambswool under the sheet. These are comfortable for the baby to sleep on, and can be machine washed, thrown into the dryer, and be back on the cradle or cot within the day!

Try not to resort to those horrible PVC-backed mattress overlays. They may be hygienic, and used in hospitals, but they don't breathe. Those of us who laid plastic under our sheets in late pregnancy, close to water-breaking time, know how uncomfortable it is!

In any case, I found my baby's underblanket was not so much a necessity, as good insurance and extra comfort. Using disposable nappies, or cloth nappies covered by pilchers, there was never any wetting of the sheets, let alone the mattress. The only moisture to seep through the sheets was dribble or milk coming up from the mouth, and that can be remedied by covering the head area of the sheet, first with a nappy, then with an empty pillowcase, bunny rug or folded sheet.

Baby bag
Choose one with lots of compartments and zipped pockets (for holding new nappies, discarded nappies, wipes, clips, tissues, creams and plastic bags). Make sure there's a plastic change mat, either attached or loose. Some have a built-in insulated polystyrene bottle holder, useful for keeping bottles of expressed milk or formula upright and cool when travelling. Many prefer to buy an ordinary carry bag rather than a baby bag, reasoning that it's cheaper, smarter, and you can choose from a more exciting colour and fabric range.

Baby capsule or car seat
This is something you have to make your own decision about, after weighing up the pros and cons. Some mothers I've met swear by convertible car seats, for 0–4 years, which are higher and shallower. They say they're much easier to get baby in and out of, they're not as hot and stuffy, and the baby gets a better view out of the window. And you don't risk strain on your back from lugging the cumbersome capsule to the car and back.

The disadvantages of the seats are that they're more expensive (although you don't then have to buy a new car seat at 6 months), they don't fit into some small cars, and you may wake up your sleeping baby while transferring him in or out of the car.

The baby capsule, on the other hand, has the big advantage of being portable, enabling you to carry a sleeping baby to and from the car without disturbing him, and it can also act as a bassinet at your destination. Also, capsules are recommended by authorities as the safest way to transport baby. You can hire one if you don't wish to outlay the purchase price.

Remember that babies shouldn't be left in capsules for more than 2 hours at a time, as it's not good for their posture or spine. Carrying baby around in a capsule is not good for your back, either, so you need to take care.

Whichever you choose, it's vital that you get the equipment installed properly by a qualified fitter. Ask your hospital for a recommendation. Different cars have different safety requirements (particularly in the case of some four-wheel drives), which you or your partner may not be aware of. It's just not worth leaving any grey areas where this is concerned. Check with the motoring authority in your state for the latest advice.

Pram/stroller
Try to find one which converts from one to the other. Find a model which has a tray below to carry shopping and baby's kit — this is invaluable. Without a tray you have to hang your bags over the handles, which can cause a dangerous imbalance (even tip the pram over), and is simply not as convenient. Also consider weight and portability. You'll spend a lot of time heaving your pram in and out of the car boot, and trying to fold and unfold it with one hand, so make sure it is easy to use. It's convenient if it can stand up on its own when folded and doesn't roll down the hill while you're putting baby in the car! And it's best if you can reverse the handle so that baby is facing you rather than facing ahead (which means you can see him as you walk).

Unless you're rich, don't buy a fancy English-style pram which doesn't convert to a stroller. In the life of the vehicle, the baby will spend more time sitting up than lying down, so you'll be grateful for a pram which you can gradually adjust to a more upright position as he learns to support himself. You can buy an English-style pram which does convert, and does have a tray, but make sure your car is big enough to fit it into the boot.

SHOPPING TIPS FOR THE FIRST 6 MONTHS

Baby pouch or sling
Pouches are just wonderful for carrying and soothing a baby for short periods (not more than 1 to 2 hours) and for use when shopping. Not everybody likes them, but it's worth borrowing one for a trial run. If you do buy one, choose a style which fully encases the baby and has a detachable dribble bib between baby's face and your chest. This protects whatever clothing you're wearing — otherwise you could be drenched within minutes if you have a baby prone to vomiting or dribbling! Make sure it's practical — easy to put baby in and adjust without help, with a wide comfortable seat and a stiff neck support (so you don't have to use your hand to support the baby's head). Most are supposed to take babies up until 6 months (after that they're too heavy anyway), but if your baby's big, like mine, you may only get 4 months' use out of it.

Baby bouncer or portable chair
There are a variety of bouncers, rockers and portable chairs on the market. Look for one you can adjust, so that baby can sit up at more of an angle as his neck strengthens. The portable chair, sometimes called a Fraser chair, is an alternative to a soft bouncer. Usually made of moulded plastic, this is more compact, gives the baby more support, and can be gradually adjusted in steepness. They're great for the early months, but stronger babies (over 4 months) can often overbalance and knock them over, so you have to take care. The moulded rocker chair is more versatile in that it can be adjusted to either rock or remain stable. For safety's sake, never sit any of these chairs on benchtops or tables.

Activity gym
This is an overhead structure with hanging baubles, attached to a colourful mat for baby to lie on at play time, all in a convenient fold-up format. They also come without the mat attachment. You probably won't use it until baby is about 2 months old, but it doesn't hurt to shop around and get a good one now. Alternatively, you can buy rattles and rings and make your own when the time comes.

Mobiles

You can hang mobiles above the cradle, to amuse at play time, and above the change table as a distraction when baby is niggly or wriggly. Wind-up musical mobiles can work magic on an unhappy baby. Colourful ones (especially those with smiling faces) are great for long-term use. For the first 2 months baby will appreciate contrast more than colour. Look out for black-and-white mobiles, or toys inspired by the movie '101 Dalmatians'.

Medical kit

At the very least, make sure you have some infant paracetamol (for bringing down a fever) and a thermometer. Plastic digital thermometers, which beep when they're ready, are easier to use and to read than traditional thin glass thermometers. They're also less fragile — but more expensive. You can now buy digital thermometers which bend to mould into the shape of baby's underarm. An even easier way to take baby's temperature is with a forehead fever thermometer, or fever strip, which you press firmly onto the forehead (after removing protective backing). The squares change colour to reveal the degree of heat. This may not be quite as accurate as conventional methods, but it's fast and practical.

Safety power points and safety switches

Both are important. Your electrician can replace your ordinary power points with safety points. This means that the slots in the socket are shut, so that no-one can poke objects into them. If all three slots are activated at once (when you put in a plug), the slots spring open. You might as well get all your power points replaced with safety ones now, if you intend to stay in your home for at least the next 12 months. In no time at all, your baby will be crawling, and it's just not worth the risk. Push-in plastic socket protectors are a much cheaper option, but it's easy to forget to replace them after using a power point. Also have the electrician install an earth leakage detector (also called a safety switch, or safety circuit breaker) if your home hasn't one already — this could save a life.

SHOPPING TIPS FOR THE FIRST 6 MONTHS

Grooming needs
Don't forget a small, soft hairbrush and some baby nail clippers or scissors. Some mothers use an emery board, but you have to be careful not to sand baby's tender skin.

Breast pump
If you're breastfeeding, you'll probably have to express milk at some time during the first 6 months — either because your breasts are too full or uncomfortable, because baby won't take the breast, or because you need milk for a babysitter or day-care centre. You may become skilled at expressing with your fingers (I wasn't), or you may be happy with one of the inexpensive plastic manual models.

If you need to express often, you'll appreciate the small battery-operated (or even electric) models which you can use with one hand. You may well chuckle now, but wait until you have hard, bloated breasts, and aching wrists from trying to rhythmically express milk with a manual pump using both hands, or have experienced the frustration of trying to manage with your fingers.

If you don't want to buy at this stage, at least check their availability with your chemist. Breast pumps can be hired from the Nursing Mothers' Association and some chemists.

Audio cassettes
Meditation music, lullaby and nursery rhyme tapes will be useful from babyhood through to preschool.

Baby book
Make certain that you have a special book or folder in which to record your baby's progress and the special events in his life. I didn't and now I regret it. It's so easy to forget what happened and when it happened. If you find the commercial books too cute, buy a beautifully bound book with blank pages, or even a plain scrapbook.

Photo album
Buy a large one with add-in pages. Believe me, you'll use every one of them (possibly in the first week)!

If I was bottlefeeding I would have bought

Bottles and teats
You'll need at least 6 glass or plastic bottles if you wish to prepare all baby's drinks for the day in advance, and leave them in the fridge. But buy more, because they're easily mislaid. It may be fun to experiment with different bottle styles, but it's more practical if you buy all the same type.

Teats come in a bewildering variety of speeds, shapes and materials. Check with your chemist, child health nurse or lactation advisor as to the best type for your particular needs.

Don't forget a good bottle brush to clean them. You can also buy a special brush for teats.

Electric bottle warmer
This is by no means necessary, but is handy and foolproof, compared with heating bottles in hot water. (Using the microwave is not recommended, as the formula continues to heat when removed, and can burn baby.)

Formula dispenser
You can buy these with three sections to hold pre-measured formula amounts. Or buy pre-measured sachets of formula — just open the sachet and add to water. Great for travelling.

Thermal bottle carrier
This keeps boiled water warm (for making up feeds while travelling) or bottles of formula cool.

Water jug
Use this for storing boiled water to mix with formula. Choose one which has a lid (and fits in the steam steriliser, if you have one).

Electric steam steriliser
This may be a luxury you can't afford, but it's the most recent and most efficient way of sterilising bottles and other equipment. You

just add water, switch on, and in a short time it switches itself off, job completed. Compare this to an hour's soaking in Milton, a chemical solution which you have to prepare, or the hassle of boiling items for 10 minutes in a saucepan. You can also buy microwave steam sterilisers, which take just 9 minutes, but at the time of writing they didn't have unanimous approval from health professionals. Check with your child health nurse as to which brand is the best option.

Luxury items (nice if you can afford them!)

Baby monitor
This is useful if you are worried you won't hear your baby when he cries. Buy one with a portable receiver that can run on batteries, and has a good transmitting range. This means you can take it with you while you hang out the washing, and still hear the baby if he so much as coughs in the nursery. (Find one which tells you when the batteries are low, and when it's out of range.) It's also useful if you visit friends, and have to leave baby in a room some distance from the noisy entertaining area.

Baby backpack
This is the next stage up from the sling. You can use a backpack as soon as baby can hold his head erect (4 to 6 months). It has a frame and a proper seat, and is usually worn happily by fathers, which gives your back a break. Great for bushwalking (but should only be used for short periods — not all day!).

Baby hammock
A comfy baby-sized hammock on its own stand. Hammocks are used in some hospitals and birth centres because they're great for soothing babies — when they move, they create their own rocking motions. Make sure that you buy one which is well ventilated — they should have mesh sides — and always ensure baby is lying on his back, so there's no chance of suffocation. Hammocks should not be used when baby is strong and mobile enough to roll out.

Baby swing
A swing on its own stand, which will both soothe and amuse. You can buy either mechanical wind-up or battery-operated models, so the baby can swing happily while you go about your chores. But, like the hammock, it's a large (and expensive) piece of play equipment, only suitable if you have enough room in your house or flat.

Portable cot
This makes life easier when you visit friends for dinner, providing a snug, safe place for baby to sleep. It's a fold-up cot made from tubular steel and vinyl, which sits on the floor like a playpen. You don't need one for a newborn but you'll appreciate it when baby's more mobile and it will last him until toddlerhood. A word of warning: don't replace the hard mattress which comes with the cot with a softer, thicker variety. Standard mattress sizes won't fit correctly, and you run the risk of baby's head becoming jammed in the gap. These have been known to collapse, and strangle or suffocate the baby inside.

Rocking chair
Maybe you can pick up a second-hand one (keep an eye out at garage sales). Not everyone agrees they're worth purchasing, but I've seen babies lulled to sleep in no time, held by a rocking mother, when all else failed. A comfortable and relaxing way to soothe your baby (that's if you can get the other members of your family off the chair!).

Dishwasher basket
Find one specifically designed to hold teats and bottle caps (for washing before sterilisation).

Clothes dryer
If you didn't have a dryer before (we didn't), you'll certainly appreciate one now. You won't believe how much washing you have, even if you don't use cloth nappies. As well as soiled baby clothes, you'll probably have to wash your own things more frequently. It's great to be able to throw clothes in the dryer and use them again the next day. Besides, you'll have precious little time to hang out washing — any time-saving device is a boon.

SHOPPING TIPS FOR THE FIRST 6 MONTHS

Video camera
A video camera is invaluable to capture hours of precious memories, and provide your baby and his future family with an irreplaceable heirloom. If you can't afford to buy one, why not try to borrow one for a weekend from a friend or family member?

Note that many of the items mentioned here have been tested by the consumer magazine *Choice*. You can back-order issues detailing the items which have passed their rigorous tests.

I wouldn't have bought

Audio-cassette of 'womb noise'
Supposedly, this is to help baby sleep! But the droning beat will drive you mad, while baby will drift off just as happily to the sound of the vacuum cleaner, or the radio!

Baby bath
They're so hard to carry and empty, you're better off using the hand basin or laundry sink (cleaned thoroughly, of course) and, later on, the big bath (with you in it as well). But if you do want to buy a bath, choose a deep one, rather than a contoured one (usually attached to a change table), which are too shallow to enable baby to float. And find one with a plug. That way you can place it on the kitchen draining board, and afterwards slide it to one side and empty it straight into the sink. Or get your partner to put a strong board over the big bath to put the baby bath on.

Nappy wipes, powder, oil, shampoo, cotton buds, and various creams in large supply
You tend to get snowed with these sorts of things later, from relatives, nappy companies and hospital gift bags, so wait and see before you splurge. In any case, many mothercraft classes tell you to clean baby only with plain water and dispense with the creams (can cause allergies) and talc (too drying). All you really need at first is a sorbolene and glycerine moisturiser or some olive oil, and some zinc

and castor oil cream or Curash powder, if baby suffers from nappy rash. I still have a shelf bulging with toiletries which have never been used.

For the hospital stay I'd have bought

For breasts

- Packet of disposable cotton breast pads. (Start with one packet, and buy more if you need them.)
- Inexpensive plastic breast pump (so you can have a practice run when your milk comes in).
- Nipple creams are no longer recommended. Rub some breastmilk on the nipple after the feed instead.

For stitches

- Hairdryer (for drying stitches after showering).
- Ultra-soft toilet paper.
- Bicarbonate of soda (a teaspoon in warm water soothes soreness and itching).
- Salt (also a good soother when added to the bath).
- Hand-held shower hose to douche stitches when you get home.

For bleeding

- Several packets (at least) of sanitary pads. Some women like maternity pads; some find them too bulky for comfort and use heavy duty pads instead (test them out before the birth). You might even appreciate some large disposable babies' nappies for the first few days when bleeding is heaviest!

For pain or discomfort

- Hospital staff can provide you with traditional pain-killing medication if necessary. But if you're into natural remedies, you may like to consult a naturopath, herbalist or health food store for a preparation which could help with postnatal discomfort.

SHOPPING TIPS FOR THE FIRST 6 MONTHS

Clothing

- Several cotton maternity bras. Have them fitted before going to hospital, but make sure there's plenty of extra room in the bra — when your milk comes in, it will suddenly fit! Don't buy too many until you start breastfeeding and can judge which style suits you best.
- Disposable underwear. Make sure the size is generous enough to accommodate large pads — a friend used her husband's old underpants instead!
- Breastfeeding garments. You'll probably be breastfeeding in front of visitors so remember that a top you can lift up is often easier and more discreet than something which buttons down the front.
- Comfortable, attractive clothes. Remember, you don't have to spend all your hospital time in pyjamas or nighties. It's good to be able to wear something relatively glamorous when you feel up to it (after all, you're now minus the huge tummy!). You may also have the opportunity to go out to dinner with your partner one evening, while your baby is cared for in the nursery.

Frozen meals

- Not for you, but for your partner! If the poor man is 'batching' while you're in hospital, he'll risk starvation, no matter how good a cook he normally is. He'll be spending every spare minute with you and the baby, often getting home late at night. And he'll be so excited, the thought of food will be far from his mind. Also freeze a few loaves of bread, and stock up on dry biscuits, cheese, tinned or packet soups, pasta sauce in jars, pasta, rice, long-life milk and pet food (for the animals, of course!).

The frozen meals will also come in handy when you and the baby arrive home. Hopefully you'll also be able to persuade some friends or relatives to cook and deliver a meal as their special treat.

BIRTH TO 1 WEEK

MILESTONES
- Cries to indicate needs.
- Startles to loud sounds (startle reflex).

WHAT THEY NEVER TELL YOU THIS WEEK

- There are many 'right' ways to care for your baby. If one expert's advice doesn't suit you, don't be afraid to seek other opinions.

- Breastfeeding may be a breeze or it may take lots of practice and be very painful or stressful. It's an art which has to be learned by both mother and baby.

- Your milk doesn't necessarily come in on day 3 or 4. It may not happen until day 5 or 6.

- Pain doesn't cease with birth: afterwards you may experience aches, soreness, stiffness, itchiness and stinging from stretching, bruising, stitches, tears, or catheter.

- Using the toilet may be painful or awkward.

- Some mothers have severe abdominal 'after birth pains' during the first week of breastfeeding, particularly if it's a second or subsequent baby.

- You will probably bleed (and maybe clot) profusely for a few days, although this doesn't always happen immediately.

- Light bleeding may continue for up to 5 or 6 weeks. (This may be more evident straight after breastfeeding, due to associated contractions of the uterus.)

- A caesarean section is major surgery, so if you have one don't expect to be springing out of bed in a hurry.

- It's okay to ban or ration visitors for the first few days if you feel you need the rest. Put yourself first.

- You can ask to leave baby in the hospital nursery at night if you desperately need some sleep.

- Although 'baby blues' traditionally happen on days 3 and 4, they may come a few days later and take you by surprise.

- From now on it will seem like an invisible cord is connecting you to your baby. You can happily while away the time gazing at him in wonder, you will be fiercely protective, and you may find it difficult, if not impossible, to be apart.

CHAPTER ONE

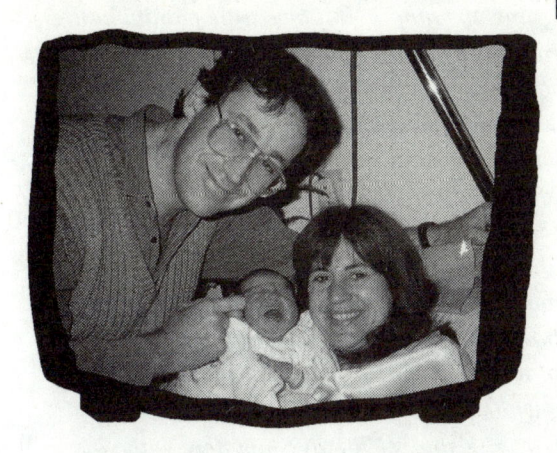

Birth to 1 week

DAY 1

6 a.m. Waaah ... waaah ... The plaintive sound penetrated my consciousness. I opened my eyes in the darkened room to see the night nurse silhouetted against the warm glow of the hallway, holding my baby in her arms. Feeding time.

I tried to move, and collapsed back onto the pillow. Pains shot through my lower body, my head throbbed, I felt woozy and overcome with exhaustion. I remembered I was attached to a drip at one end and a catheter at the other. I'd had a caesarean. A trapeze bar hung above my head for me to heave myself up with. My mouth was dry.

The nurse placed the baby in its bassinet by my bed while she helped me struggle higher up onto the pillow. I felt like a dead weight. It was agony to move. We enlisted the aid of another nurse, and together they hauled me into sitting position.

This would be the second time I'd fed our baby. The first feed was at midnight, shortly after delivery. Then they had taken him off to the night nursery. But that's all a blur. Now they gave him to me, wrapped up tightly in his blue bunny rug like a spring roll, his little red face crinkled with a wail of hunger.

One of the nurses helped me attach him to the breast. First I had to squeeze out a drop of colostrum, so he could taste this as I pressed his mouth against the nipple. It took a little manipulating. I felt lost and awkward, trying to work out hand and arm positions, but the baby seemed to know what to do. Thank goodness. It was all so strange and new to me! It was a funny sensation, like a tiny mouse gnawing at my nipple, an itch that you want to idly brush away, yet quite pleasant.

The nurse stayed with me, chatting encouragingly, and helped me take the baby off the first breast after about 15 minutes. What suction he had! We had to prise him off like a limpet, forcing a little finger into the side of his mouth to break his grip. After he'd finished on the second breast she burped him for me, and tucked him into the bassinet, while I collapsed back on the pillows, exhausted. 'He's asleep', she said. 'I'll leave him here with you now if you like.'

How exciting! I was to keep the baby here in the room, all to myself! I watched the golden morning light filter through the curtains, and thought blissfully about the whole new life that lay ahead.

Your baby this week

Your baby is just gorgeous, although on arrival he may not look like your vision of a porcelain doll. His head may be elongated, he may be wrinkly, blotchy, bald, bruised or bloodshot, depending on the type of birth. But rest assured, babies even out and blossom very quickly. His fingernails may be long (and already need trimming), and his skin may look as though he's been in the bath too long. He may weigh more or less than the average 3.4 kilograms ($7\frac{1}{2}$ pounds).

If you're in hospital this week, your baby will not be dressed in the pretty clothes you've bought, but in plain hospital gear, unless you can persuade staff otherwise. He'll be wrapped rather tightly in a bunny rug, to give him the same feeling of security he had in the womb. And he'll probably be placed on his back to sleep, in keeping with the latest findings regarding risk of cot death.

Make the most of the first week

For most of us, the first 5 days or so is spent either in hospital or at a birthing centre. Make the most of this relatively luxurious period, when you're still in a state of post-birth bliss, your family and friends are gathering around you to celebrate, you are waited on, fed three nutritious meals a day, there's no housework or washing of nappies, and you have staff at hand to help you settle into a good feeding routine.

Take advantage of this time to learn as much as you can about baby care since this is the best chance you'll have to get intensive input from trained staff.

If you choose the option of an early discharge program offered by many hospitals (where a midwife comes to visit you at home daily until about day 7), make sure you go home to rest, rather than try to take up normal household duties. And organise a visit to your child health centre as soon as possible.

Relish the moment

This may seem obvious, but snatch the moment — when you and your partner are both elated, and you in particular are experiencing that heady mixture of joy, relief and wellbeing that usually follows birth — to have your family celebration in whatever form is right for you. We had expensive champagne ready on ice, but after a long labour followed by a caesarean, I wasn't up to drinking it (a cup of tea was more my speed, and it mixed better with the painkillers!). Whether you have a quiet and tender party for three, or a jovial champagne gathering of friends and relatives in the delivery suite, take advantage of this emotionally charged period, because you'll never get another high like it.

Hospital tips

- Ask questions. Write them down when they occur to you and save them up for later. And even write down the answers — it's surprising how easy it is to forget!

- Attend maternity ward classes — bathing, baby massage, breastfeeding — where possible, as practical demonstrations are invaluable. (Expect to miss out on some because of baby crying or feeding, or because you need to sleep.)

- Don't be afraid to ask. If something puzzles you, seek opinions from every nurse, doctor or expert you come across. Opinions often differ, especially with breastfeeding, and advice from someone else may suit you better.

- If you're having trouble with breastfeeding, cry for help immediately — don't be shy. It's vital for baby and mother to learn correct attachment from the very beginning. Delaying may make the problem worse, and turn you off breastfeeding for life!

- Ask if your hospital has a lactation consultant or child health nurse available for a one-to-one session.

- Try to schedule your first baby bathing session at a time when dad can be present.

- Take a few moments to read all leaflets which come your way, and start digesting the first chapters of your baby-care books. There'll be precious little time for this when you get home.

- Be assertive and don't let yourself be bullied. Always remember that it's *your* baby, and it's you and your baby who have to be happy. New parents sometimes find hospital staff intimidating. They feel the midwife or nurse must always be right. She may be but, on the other hand, she may just have a different set of priorities. Don't be afraid to stick up for what you believe is right for you.

DAY 1

8 a.m. The slightest movement of my lower body hurt. The painkiller they'd given me during the night (after assuring me that it wouldn't adversely affect the baby through my colostrum) had worn off, but I was reluctant to take another dose.

Nurses bustled in and out, giving me a body wash, a fresh sanitary pad (you bleed for several days, sometimes even longer, whether you've had a caesarean or not), and taking my temperature and blood pressure. The baby lay peaceful and still, hidden from view under his cotton blanket.

No sooner had I drifted off to sleep than there was a brisk knock on the door, and my obstetrician breezed in, looking disgustingly well-groomed and chirpy for 8 a.m. To think she had delivered this baby only 9 or 10 hours ago.

'How are we today?' Cynthia asked, looking rather pleased with herself.

I smiled wanly. How did I look! I certainly hadn't expected to be laid up like this after having the baby. Caesarean or not. I remember visiting my sister-in-law in hospital 2 years ago, after her baby had been delivered by caesarean, and being surprised at how pale and weak she was, lying there attached to a drip. I hadn't realised this was run-of-the-mill. No-one mentions before the event that having a caesarean is really major surgery!

Cynthia examined my scar, told me everything was terrific, and was out the door before I had time to collect my thoughts. I remembered that she had to finish her rounds here at the hospital and be in her rooms by 9 a.m. for appointments. In her wake the paediatrician bounced in, resplendent in yellow polka-dot bow tie. What a circus! The baby was pronounced fine. Then someone brought me a welcome cup of tea (at least I could drink) and the cleaners came in to vacuum. Phew! What a busy day — and only just past 9 a.m.

A soft knock on the door heralded the arrival of a fieldful of daffodils, with Tristan in tow. What extravagance! He knows they're my favourite flowers — how fortunate they're in season. Mixed with the glorious sheafs of yellow were other assorted bunches, blue and white. Suddenly, it was spring.

The hospital routine

The hospital stay does have its drawbacks, one of which is that you have to follow their routine, as well as the baby's. And that, it seems, means constant interruptions. A night punctuated by nurses thrusting a crying baby at your breast, or offering painkillers if you've had a caesarean. Staff bustling in and out from dawn to help you wash, change your bed, give you fresh sanitary pads, take your temperature and blood pressure, tell you what's on today, offer solace, religious advice or newspapers, wheel in breakfast. Just as you think you'll get a break, the cleaners zoom in with the vacuum, other staff refresh the flowers, clean the bathroom and take your menu selection. Then there's the obstetrician, the paediatrician, a florist delivery, a nurse with forms to fill in. Yet another knock on the door, this time your partner — and you realise, with some surprise, that it's still early morning!

At least most hospitals have a 'quiet time' — a few hours, usually after lunch, dedicated to rest for you and the baby. Visitors are usually forbidden, and phone calls not put through. Make the most of this sanctuary of uninterrupted peace, and make sure that everyone, even your partner, respects it. This sets a good pattern for when you arrive home.

Visitors

When you want visitors depends on how you feel and how social an animal you are. But be warned, you may prefer to reserve the first few days just for yourself, your partner and your immediate family.

Be sure to put your own needs first. If you don't feel like seeing even close friends for a while, leave a message with the hospital switchboard, telling them when you'll be ready to receive visitors. People usually ring before coming. You may like to specify they come within certain visiting hours. Or ask your partner to tell them when would be a good time to visit. There's nothing worse than having someone 'pop in' on you when you're half naked and struggling awkwardly with a dirty nappy, or dissolved in tears, trying vainly to attach a screaming newborn to your breast.

Telephone tactics

If you have a room with a private phone, it's a good idea not to give your direct number to anyone except your partner, and perhaps immediate family members or close friends.

If people have to come through the switchboard to speak to you, you're more in control — it means you can hold calls when you need a rest, and you won't be accidentally disturbed during quiet time. (Remember to tell those who have your direct number not to call during quiet-time hours.) There are other times during the hectic hospital and baby-minding schedule that you'll be absolutely desperate for a nap, and if you can ask the switchboard to hold all calls until further notice, you'll avoid being woken by Aunt Daphne, who's dying to find out every last detail of the birth.

Some women take the phone off the hook as a last resort — but this could frustrate the switchboard, not to mention the dedicated daddy trying to get through in his coffee break.

Rooming-in

This means having the baby with you in your room at all times. Most hospitals now encourage rooming-in so that you get to know your baby during your short stay. However, your innocent, idealistic plans to room-in may change abruptly once baby arrives. When you're lying sore and exhausted (albeit elated), and desperately in need of sleep, a nurse's offer to take the baby into the nursery for the night may be hard to resist, despite your earlier resolve never to let the precious thing out of your sight. If you do have this opportunity, don't feel guilty — after all, night nurses can sleep during the day, and are well-qualified to take good care of your baby.

Swaddling

It used to worry me that the nurses wrapped my baby so firmly in his blanket to put him to sleep, pinning his arms across his chest. What if he had an itchy nose? They said that there were good reasons for swaddling: it makes babies feel more secure, because they have been so closely contained in the uterus, and actually lowers their heart rate; it helps keep them warm; and it helps control involuntary movements, such as arms flailing out, avoiding the risk of hitting or scratching themselves in the face while asleep.

However, because of the risk of SIDS (see page 66), many child health nurses now advise against the traditional practice of swaddling, unless baby is very unsettled. They recommend dressing baby warmly instead, and just lightly wrapping him in a cotton sheet for the first few weeks. Warm baths and cuddling are often encouraged as good settling techniques.

Your body

You'll be elated all week (at least until about day 4 when the 'baby blues' may hit), and unable to believe quite how you managed such a feat. At the same time, you'll be either tired or utterly exhausted; and, depending on your mode of delivery, will probably be suffering some form of discomfort.

Post-vaginal birth
You'll have soreness from vaginal bruising, tears or stitches. If you've had an episiotomy, it might be agony to sit down or urinate. As the tissues heal, you'll have to deal with itching as well as the stinging. You may be too terrified to use your bowels. Talk to a nurse about what to do, rather than suffering in silence and frustration.

Post-caesarean birth
They never tell you before the event that having a caesarean is major surgery, and you're not going to be bouncing out of bed for some time. You'll probably have a drip at one end, and a catheter at the other, taking no solid food for a day or two. Expect to feel very sore and sorry for yourself. Because so much muscle tissue has been cut, it's especially important to begin a mild exercise routine from the first week — even though it's the last thing you'll feel like — and to walk upright (when you can walk), rather than bent forward at the waist.

Bleeding

You can expect heavy bleeding for at least a few days (maybe with clotting), and continued light bleeding for a few weeks. You may even have a slight discharge for up to 5 or 6 weeks (but consult a doctor if you have prolonged heavy bleeding). Don't use tampons, as they can cause infection while the cervix is closing and the uterus is returning to normal position. Use either maternity pads or heavy-duty pads, with disposable pants. You may need more than the 2 packs most people advise. I know several women who had to resort to wearing large disposable babies' nappies for the first few days because bleeding was so heavy!

After-birth pains

You may experience abdominal pain during the first week of breastfeeding, during or straight after the feed (although it is more common if this is not your first baby). The hormone which controls milk 'let down' (oxytocin) also controls the contraction and shrinking of the uterus. The cramps may be extreme enough to require pain killers (some women compare them to labour pains) or it may feel like your tummy's being vacuumed in, in rhythm to the baby's sucking. They usually ease after the first few feeds, and disappear by the end of the week. You may like to try herbal preparations to get some relief, rather than traditional painkillers.

Post-episiotomy tips

- Douche stitches externally with a hand-held shower several times a day.
- When urinating, lean forward (even put your hands on the floor) so that urine does not flow back onto stitches.
- Dissolve several tablespoons of bicarbonate of soda or salt in a bowl of lukewarm water, and sit in this after passing urine. Works wonders for stinging, itching and discomfort and the solution is also good for nipples.

- Use your own ultra-soft toilet paper.
- Pat stitches dry first, then use hairdryer (not too close).
- Ask staff for an 'ice finger' (which is like a thin cold-pack) or try an icypole (in wrapper) between your legs. Insert inside sleeve of the pad to hold it in place.
- Dab on witch-hazel (available from the chemist).
- Drink lots of soda water which makes the urine less acidic and less painful to pass.
- Ask for prunes or a mild laxative if needed to help the first bowel movements.
- Sit on an inflated rubber ring. These are usually provided by the hospital but you can make your own out of foam rubber.

The first breastfeed

Feeding is usually your very first 'chore' as a new mother. Sometimes the baby will be put to your breast 5 to 10 minutes after birth or (particularly after a caesarean) he may be taken away for weighing, health checks and a bath, before being brought to your bedside half an hour later.

You probably expected to have plump breasts full of creamy white milk to offer your newborn but feeding doesn't mean milk until a few days after the event. What your breasts are producing at this stage is colostrum. You'll need to squeeze out a drop or two in order to interest baby in the prospect of a first meal. Then stroke the cheek nearest your breast so that he turns and opens his mouth (the 'rooting reflex'), and press his mouth against the nipple until he starts sucking. It may feel a little awkward at first, trying to sort out where to put your hands and arms, but with any luck the baby will know what to do and suck on, regardless of your discomfort. (Like learning how to drive a car, when you haven't done it before, it can be quite a task coordinating all the movements!)

BIRTH TO 1 WEEK

At best, breastfeeding can be a mild, funny and quite pleasant sensation; at worst it can be extremely painful, possibly meaning baby's mouth is not properly covering the whole nipple. You may be surprised at the strength of that little mouth, which can grip you like a limpet and be almost impossible to dislodge until you get the knack! Sometimes you'll have to ease your little finger into the side of his mouth to break the grip. Then it's time to try the next breast. The first round of breastfeeding will most likely leave you exhausted, and ready for a sleep yourself (as if you weren't beforehand, after all that labour!).

What is colostrum?

Colostrum is a clear or yellowish fluid produced by your breasts during the last few months of pregnancy and for a few days after the birth, before the milk 'comes in'. Some nurses call it 'liquid gold'. Rich in protein, nutrients and valuable antibodies, it's all the food your baby needs for the first few days.

If you and your baby are separated for any reason after birth, ask if you can express colostrum to feed him in your absence.

Breastfeeding difficulties

In an ideal situation the baby senses the breast and immediately knows what to do, latches on, and begins to feed hungrily, while you provide the correct support without undue body distortion and make sure he is not feeding in a way which will cause your nipples pain, now or later.

Unfortunately, not all babies are born accomplished suckers, and not all of us will have this trouble-free experience. While I found the initial sensation of breastfeeding rather pleasant, another mother told me she felt as if razor blades were ripping at her breasts, despite the fact that she had prepared and manipulated her nipples religiously during late pregnancy. Babies actually have a chewing motion, so depending on your baby's gums and technique, the effects can be harsh.

Experts now stress that the most important aspect is 'attaching' (also called 'latching on'). If baby is not correctly attached from the very beginning (with his mouth opened wide to cover the whole nipple and areola), there are likely to be problems. What they don't tell you is that even if baby is correctly attached, there may still be some pain.

It's important to ask for help for the first few feeds at least. If you start off on the right foot, there's a good chance things will continue without a hitch.

For some women, their problems are exacerbated by what they see as unsympathetic, brusque or even aggressive methods of assistance from midwives or hospital staff. They may feel they're being treated roughly, as a 'piece of flesh'. It may simply be that the hospital is busy or understaffed or that your nurse has other priorities. First-time mothers (and fathers as well) are in a vulnerable position, and easily intimidated by the bustling efficiency and authority of some nurses. Ask for help. Feel confident about standing up for yourself, and speaking out if you're dissatisfied. If you have a personality clash with your advisor, 'latch on' to another one!

At least during these first few days you have the support and assistance of a health care team. So, make every effort to get breastfeeding well established before you go home! If not, speak to the hospital's lactation specialist about other options. Maybe you could return to her for a visit, book a lactation expert to come to your home, go on to a private hospital which offers postnatal care, spend a day at a family care cottage, or risk the wrath of the midwives by doing a crash course in bottlefeeding, just in case.

Frequency of feeding

During the first few days, your baby isn't in desperate need of nutrition. He lives off the fat he was born with. In fact, most babies lose weight during the first week (up to 10 per cent of their birth weight) because of the passing of meconium and the small milk intake. He will start to put on weight after your milk has come in, and will probably regain his birth weight by 7 to 10 days.

How frequently they demand feeding varies greatly from baby to baby. We felt fortunate in that our baby fed only every 6 hours for the first few days, tending to sleep rather than eat after the stress of being born. Other babies may demand food every 2 or 3 hours.

To avoid confusion, remember that when people speak of time between feeds, they mean the time elapsed between beginning (not finishing) one feed and beginning another. So feeding at 2 p.m., 5 p.m., 8 p.m. and so on, means you're feeding at 3-hour intervals (although it's rare that feeding patterns are this precise!).

Babies who are being bottlefed will take only a small amount this week — about 60 ml per kilogram of body weight per day, graduating to about 150 ml per kilogram by next week.

DAY 2

Hooray! The drip and catheter were removed this morning, and I was able to have my first shower and shampoo. Bliss! Felt much more normal although I'm still shuffling around stooped over like an old lady, because of my sore abdomen. Afterwards I stretched out on a comfy chair in the nursery (where baby was still asleep, after only one feed during the night) and basked topless in the warm late-winter sunshine streaming in through the window. It's a favourite spot for feeding mums, as moderate exposure to sunlight and plenty of air helps heal nipples and make them supple. I noticed I had a slight blister appearing. Must be sure to stick to the correct breast-care routine.

This afternoon I lay back on my pillows with a cup of tea, surrounded by sweet-smelling flowers, the baby sleeping beside my bed, and let out a long sigh of satisfaction and relief. It was as if I'd been standing for ages in a long queue, and finally reached the end. I had arrived!

Caring for baby

Meconium
For the first day or two, baby will pass meconium, a greenish-black substance which needs to be eliminated before normal bowel actions occur.

Wet nappies
He should have 6 to 8 a day when feeding properly. However, nappy wash services often quote up to 10 nappies a day, just to be on the safe side.

Lifting
Take care, and remind your partner, to support the back of baby's neck while lifting and carrying, until he develops some strength in his neck muscles (at least 6 weeks).

Navels
Most hospitals recommend simply cleaning the navel with water or saline solution (it used to be methylated spirits), and drying with a cotton bud, until it shrivels and drops off naturally.

Nails
If fingernails or toenails need trimming, the nurse may suggest peeling off the soft nail tips with your fingers or teeth. The mere idea sent shivers down my spine so I preferred to buy round-tipped baby scissors to carefully do the job. A paper emery board is sometimes suggested, but there's a risk of sanding off baby's delicate skin.

DAY 3

I'm feeling terrific. My milk has come in, so my breasts are very large, but not too uncomfortable — yet. I'm finally managing to walk with a straight back, after the caesarean. And, for the first time, I've been able to get the baby onto the breast myself, change, burp and put him to sleep, without any help. What a sense of achievement!

Another first has been eye-to-eye contact with the baby. Until now, it's been just sleep, feed, sleep. But this evening, after his feed, Tristan and I concentrated on getting his attention, and he actually looked at us both in turn for about half an hour. How exciting! We really felt we were communicating.

After poring over baby books we've decided that the only boy's name we really like is the one we thought of before the birth — Rupert. Reminiscent of things English (like his father) and Rupert Bear books (which Tristan read as a child), it seems to suit him. We've written Rupert on the bassinet tag but we've decided to harbour the secret for a while and try the name out ourselves before officially notifying the outside world.

Naming baby

If the baby arrives before you've agreed on a name, don't panic. While many people bestow their favourite name while the baby's in the womb (or even before conception), there are some who prefer to wait a while and get to know the baby before finding a name that fits. Don't be bullied by family or nursing staff — after all, you and your child have to live with it for a long time!

Remember to register the name with Births, Deaths and Marriages. You have at least a few weeks to do this (the number of days differs from state to state). As soon as you can, have the baby's name added to your Medicare card, in case you have to take him to a doctor in the first few weeks. Some hospitals will help you arrange this.

When your milk comes in

Just when you think you've got everything under control (or it couldn't get any worse!), your milk will arrive, and it's a whole new ball game. Usually around day 3 or 4 (but sometimes as early as day 1 or 2, sometimes day 5 or 6), your breasts will suddenly swell to the size and consistency of solid melons, and the baby may have trouble even finding your nipple, let alone latching on. In the worse cases, it's like trying to suck the side of a taut balloon!

Don't be disillusioned if at first you don't succeed. Maybe you need to express a little milk before each feed, so the nipple is softer for baby to latch onto. It's important to remember that there are many tricks and techniques for breastfeeding, and each carer has her own particular favourite. If your first coach doesn't help you achieve success with her suggested techniques, don't be afraid to ask another nurse for help next time, or call for a specialist. It's not worth suffering in order not to offend anybody.

Apart from you and the baby having to cope with your newly swollen breasts, you may find feeding patterns become more frequent, or totally unpredictable.

If you leave hospital before your milk comes in, you could be in for a shock when it happens, especially if baby becomes very unsettled. Ring someone if you can't cope. Sometimes it's enough just to be reassured that this is normal.

If your milk doesn't come in

Don't panic if your milk hasn't come in by day 4. Sometimes it can take until day 5 or 6, especially if you are recovering from a difficult delivery, a large blood loss or general physical strain. If your milk is not in, then the baby will usually want to feed quite frequently, which is good, as this should encourage the milk supply to increase.

In extreme cases, when frequent feeding doesn't lead to more milk, nurses may suggest that baby's feeds be supplemented with small portions of formula. This will take the pressure off you, and keep baby happy.

In such cases, some hospitals use a technique called 'supply-line feeding'. This involves attaching a thin line, or tube, into the bottle of formula, and taping the other end to mum's nipple, while a nurse stands by to hold up the bottle. The baby is put to the breast to suck, and receives the formula instead (sneaky). Baby gets the breast and the comfort — and the sucking helps stimulate your breastmilk. Not all nurses and midwives are aware of this technique, so if you do have to resort to supplementary feeding, it may pay to ask around.

Let down

This is the funny tingling feeling in your breast either just before or just after baby starts feeding. It signifies the release of the hormone oxytocin — stimulated by baby's sucking, or by anticipation or thoughts of the baby — which contracts the milk sacs, and lets the milk down from the breast to the nipple. Suddenly, milk becomes plentiful, and feeding (or expressing) much easier. Some women never feel the let down, but continue to feed effectively.

Breastfeeding hotlines

- Contact the hospital's lactation consultant. They specialise in this area, and their role is to help women with breastfeeding problems. They can work miracles on the spot.

- Another lifesaver is the NMAA (Nursing Mothers' Association of Australia). You can telephone at any time to speak to an experienced breastfeeding mother (there's always a member rostered on during the night to take urgent calls) and they have regular meetings which you can attend before and after the birth.

- Many family care organisations also have 24-hour hotlines which you can call for advice at no charge. (See Help lines, pages 238–41.)

Turning to the bottle

Some mothers either can't, or don't want to, breastfeed for various reasons, and may decide on formula either from the very beginning, or after the first few days. Because of the nutritional benefits of breastfeeding, as well as its many other advantages, women are usually advised to persevere if milk is scarce, or feeding is painful at first. Breastfeeding often takes 4 to 6 weeks to establish and feel comfortable, so it's good if you can ride out any difficult periods.

However, if you feel very strongly that you don't want to continue, you shouldn't feel guilty. What they don't tell you is that breastfeeding, although wonderful and highly recommended, isn't necessarily right for everyone. And it won't be such a tragedy if you are unable to feed. Some doctors believe that the formulas available these days are almost as nourishing as breastmilk, and that as long as you give your baby lots of warmth and cuddles, he won't be sold short. A happy mother and baby is the most important thing.

Having said that, remember that in most cases perseverance does seem to pay off, so give it a fair go. The first 3 months are said to be the most important as far as boosting baby's immune system. At the very least, try to give baby the benefit of the colostrum (with its valuable antibodies) which is produced during the first few days.

If you're in doubt about your ability to feed adequately, or too stressed out from the attempts, seek advice from one of the experts. And if that doesn't work, call in another expert! They all seem to have different opinions, and not everyone knows what's best for you and your baby. It's no good continuing to feel miserable, or having a baby not thriving. If, for example, you have little or no milk, formula feeding may be the only option. It's not the end of the world — many of us survived with formula alone!

Even if you've no intention of ever turning to the bottle, it's a good idea to pick up a few tips on how it's done while you're there with the experts. There's a whole new world of sterilisation, powder mixing, teats and temperature testing, which is worth knowing in case you're suddenly caught out. There may come a time when your breasts are just too sore to feed, or when you feel your baby isn't getting enough breastmilk. Professional advice may well solve these problems, but it's wise to have a bottle, some formula, and the right equipment at home, just in case.

(See Baby shopping tips, pages 18–19 and Bottlefeeding, pages 83–86.)

DAY 4

The fourth day is traditionally 'baby blues' day. I woke up expecting to feel quite miserable, but surprisingly I was still feeling great, and rather smug to boot. I was now feeding in an armchair (rather than propped up in bed), resting my feet on two telephone books in order to keep my back straight. We'd settled into a routine of 6 feeds a day, about 4 hours apart. I had plenty of milk, and the baby was feeding well. By now the nurses were leaving me pretty much alone, as I had no trouble putting him to the breast myself. I knew I wasn't going to succumb to weepiness — how could it be possible when everything was going so wonderfully?

But how quickly things can change! The 7 p.m. feed went for a gruelling 1 hour (twice as long as usual), with 30 minutes at each breast. Followed by 2 hours of wind, crying and dirty nappies. I felt helpless, frustrated and exhausted. When Rupert finally fell asleep at 10 p.m. it was only to wake again at 11.45 p.m. and demand more.

By this time Tristan had gone home to bed. I rang him in a terrible state and burst into tears. The darling reappeared in my room 15 minutes later in response to the unspoken SOS, and stayed while I fed for another half-hour, fetching me tea and giving lots of comfort. Heavens, what was happening?

Baby blues

Just when you think you're going to avoid them (having told yourself that you're not going to be one to succumb), they'll hit you and have you wailing on the phone to your partner, mother or nurse. (Best to warn partners in advance!) Somehow it's not much comfort to know that this state is perfectly normal and transitory (usually only a day or two). Just weather it as best you can.

Most women seem to get the blues on day 3 or 4, but it could happen later. Think yourself lucky if you have them in hospital — it's better than at home by yourself! And if they fall on the day you leave hospital, they can really ruin your homecoming.

The cause seems to be a combination of hormonal changes, birth trauma, emotional letdown after the initial prolonged high, and utter exhaustion from exertion and lack of sleep. Mind you, the baby blues are different for everyone. Some women feel anxious or tense, some feel weepy and despairing, others just feel tired and washed out. About 30 per cent of new mums escape the blues altogether.

If you have blues that don't go away after a couple of weeks, then consult a professional. You may be suffering from postnatal depression, a condition which can, and should, be treated (see pages 188–9).

DAY 5

By now my breasts were so swollen with milk that the nipple seemed to have disappeared, and the baby was having difficulty latching on. The more he tried, the more frustrated and hungry he got; the more he cried, the more I cried, and so it went on. Finally one of the nurses showed me how to use a breast pump to express some of the excess milk, which I did very awkwardly. It improved things initially, but still the baby kept slipping off the nipple. The next nurse on duty didn't have any further advice to offer. My mood changed to anger. Why couldn't anyone help?

By midday I was a total wreck, reduced to a sobbing blob alone in my room, feeling a failure as a mother, abandoned by everyone. I warned the switchboard operator not to allow visitors, and tried to pull myself together. There must be someone I could turn to. Then I remembered kindly Sister Jan, the lactation nurse who had run the prenatal mothercraft classes at the hospital. In desperation I had her paged, and after what seemed an eternity (about 5 minutes, actually) she returned the call. I dissolved into tears again at the sound of her voice, and bleated out my dilemma. She promised she would be here within half an hour.

Ah, the relief when that woman entered my room! With one glance she had taken it all in — the tearful swollen-eyed mum crouched in a chair, the howling infant clutched to her bosom. She'd seen it all so many times before. A few swift steps and she was at my side. She spoke softly, reassuringly, as she gently rearranged my position, guided the baby's head firmly towards my nipple, and with one deft movement had him attached and happily sucking. I couldn't believe it. All those hours of trauma and now sudden peace and satisfaction. She was a miracle worker!

Sister Jan set about showing me her secrets. First, a different way of holding the baby — using the left hand to cup the left breast, and the right hand to grasp the back of the baby's head and manoeuvre it into position. This was the direct opposite of what I'd been taught, and what was illustrated in all the books, but she explained it was a good method for beginners, because using your right, rather than left hand, to position baby's head makes for much better control. I could relax into a more comfortable position when the baby was happily feeding.

She also showed me how to use two fingers either side of the nipple, to squeeze the breast into a flattened 'biscuit' shape, so the baby can latch on more easily (especially useful if the breast is really full). And she advised to get into the habit of always offering the second breast, even if you think the baby has had enough at the first.

Sister Jan walked out leaving me smiling in gratitude. She was a saint. That afternoon saw the end of our predictable feeding routine, with the baby now sometimes demanding another feed just an hour after finishing the last. The books don't warn you this might happen! But somehow I coped. If this was the baby blues, I'd been through them ... and I'll never be smug again!

Sore nipples

No matter how hard you try, or how well you've prepared, it's difficult to avoid some repercussions of baby's greedy assault on your breasts. Even if the first day or two seem painless, watch carefully for signs of blistering or cracking. With proper breast care and a little luck, you can avoid the situation where your breasts are so sore you want to give up.

If you do get a crack, seek help immediately. Don't let it get worse, because you may have to stop feeding altogether. You may be advised to 'rest and express' (that is, stop breastfeeding for a short time and express milk to feed baby instead).

Sore shoulders

Women can find themselves in all sorts of awkward positions while learning how to breastfeed — and then be too scared to move, in case the baby is dislodged! It's a posture that's new to your body and, as with any new form of exercise, you'll be putting strain on muscles you didn't realise existed. You may hunch your shoulders for prolonged periods while cradling the baby at your breast, or end up with a stiff and sore neck from gazing down at him the whole time he's feeding.

Have your feeding posture checked, making certain your back is straight and you're well supported. Make a conscious effort to relax your body and avoid locking into any one position for too long. And don't suffer in silence — try contacting the physiotherapy department at your hospital, if there is one. You may find yourself treated to a relaxing massage, which will melt all those knots away.

Tips for breast care

- Make sure the baby is correctly attached, with top and bottom lips pursed out in a K shape, so the mouth covers the whole nipple and areola. You'll know he's correctly attached if it feels comfortable, the baby has a good mouthful of breast, and when he comes off, the nipple doesn't look flattened or pinched.

- Straight after feeding, squeeze out a drop or two of the rich breastmilk, and spread gently over the nipple area (its natural antibodies help protect and heal).

- Air dry nipples if possible. Try leaving the flaps of your bra open to help healing — this is comfortable for some women, but not for others. You can try using a hairdryer to speed drying, but don't put it too close, and don't overdry, or it will be counterproductive.

- Expose nipples to mild sunlight for short intervals (3 to 5 minutes) if convenient. As well as drying excess moisture, the ultraviolet light toughens nipples and helps in the healing process.

- Current breastfeeding policy advises no use of creams of any kind (although previously paw paw cream or sorbolene and glycerine were popular to moisturise, heal and protect).
- Use cotton bras and pads — avoid anything synthetic which might irritate.
- Change breast pads frequently to avoid wetness on your skin.
- Cold cabbage leaves (from the fridge) inside your bra will relieve the heat and swelling when your milk comes in. Leave them on for about 20 minutes or until they become warm, then repeat. It may sound like an unlikely and old-fashioned remedy but, believe me, it works. Some hospitals are now wary of cabbage leaves because of the fear of insecticides (find organic cabbages). Others warn that extended use of the leaves can lead to reduced milk supply.
- Packets of frozen peas are great to use as cold packs when you're home.
- Hot packs, hot face washers (or nappies) or a hot shower will relieve engorged breasts before feeding, help start the milk flowing and make nipples softer for baby to attach.
- If your nipples become sore or cracked, you may benefit from soft silicone nipple shields which help to reduce the pain while breastfeeding and allow healing. But while they work well for some women, others find them unhelpful, too much of a bother or more trouble than they're worth. Consult your nurse or midwife first. (See Cracked or bleeding nipples, pages 45–7 and Breastfeeding tips, pages 77–8.)

Breast pumps

It's worth finding out how to use one while you're in hospital, so you're familiar with the routine if or when the need arises. You may be able to master the hand technique of expressing (I couldn't!), but many breastfeeding mothers find it quicker and easier to use a pump.

During the first few weeks, when your breasts are in this bulging condition, it's often necessary to express some milk just before feeding, to make it easier for the baby to latch on, or to relieve swelling for your own comfort. Or you may need to express after a feed, if the baby feeds from just one breast and the other becomes hard and painful.

Some mothers are forced to express for a while, because their nipples become too cracked to feed without pain or bleeding. The skill will also come in handy later on, if you need to express a bottle of milk for your partner or baby-sitter to feed in your absence, or if you plan to combine work and breastfeeding.

There are many different types of pumps, ranging from the simple manual and more efficient battery-operated ones you can find in the chemist, to the larger electric models which you can hire. The cheaper plastic manual models are effective enough, especially if they have side measurements in millilitres, and a screw top and teat for storage of milk and feeding. But depending on the model, manual expressing can be a real strain on your hands (as I found out).

A friend told me she would have given up breastfeeding altogether had she not discovered the small battery-operated breast pumps, which can be used with one hand and work like a dream. Apart from the efficiency of operation, it saved her hands the stiffness caused by pumping manually. And the single-handed operation meant she could read, talk on the phone or even feed the baby from the other breast at the same time as she expressed. Worth its weight in gold!

Alternatively, you can hire an electric pump from the Nursing Mothers' Association and some chemists. (See Expressing, pages 142–5.)

Crying tips

- During the first week, there's so much to learn and digest that you don't need extra complications, like constant wailing.
- Try feeding first (even if it seems to you he could not possibly be hungry again).

- Wet or dirty nappy is the other obvious checkpoint.
- Try putting your little finger in baby's mouth, and let him suck vigorously on that as a pacifier.
- Try putting baby's own fingers in his mouth.
- Wrap baby well, and hold him tightly against your chest, or over your shoulder, patting and rocking rhythmically.
- Put baby in the bassinet, and pat him slowly and rhythmically on his back (mimicking the sound of mother's heartbeat heard in the womb).
- Sing a lullaby or nursery rhyme (you may need to do some quick research!).
- Find some soothing music on the radio.
- Give baby a deep warm bath.
- Hand baby to someone else to give yourself a break before trying some of these techniques again.
- If none of the above work, there is a last resort — the dummy.

Dummies

You may have sworn never to use one, but by the time day 2 or 3 of crying dawns you may change your mind, and reason that your mental and physical health is worth it! Many of us have been frightened off dummies by stories of teeth being deformed, or fear they'll still be using a dummy at 4 (years, that is). But what they don't tell you is that anything within reason that will stop a crying baby crying, and give you some peace and comfort in the initial stages, has its place. In fact, some babies have a greater sucking need than others, and will suck at the breast for ages, even if no longer hungry. Dummies are often advised for this type of baby. But don't take it for granted that your baby will take to a dummy. He may well object to this foreign object, and spit it out.

You can always wean off the dummy at a later stage (say around 3 months, or when they start on solids at 4 or 5 months). But don't give it to baby as a matter of habit, only as part of a settling technique. And take it out after he's gone to sleep.

DAY 6

The sun was shining, and I felt great. Scrambled out of bed at 7.30 a.m., before the baby woke up, and showered and shampooed my hair. I was ravenous but, unfortunately, so was the baby. He opened his eyes just as my breakfast tray arrived, and insisted on having his meal first: half an hour on one breast and burping time and 15 minutes on the second breast and burping time, then nappy time ... One and a half hours later, cold leathery scrambled eggs had never tasted so good!

It's just dawned on me that life is not going to be as easy as I'd thought. He dictates the schedule. That means if I arrange anything for a specific time, and the baby decides he's hungry at that moment, I have no choice but to sit down and breastfeed. I've already missed my first hospital postnatal exercise class for this very reason. Hmm, I guess he'll settle into a routine soon.

Nappies

Don't worry if you can't get the hang of those safety pins while you're in hospital. Some women seem to have the knack while others (like me) fasten nappies so inadequately that they're down around the baby's knees in no time. Fortunately, there is now a better way (apart from disposables!). Plastic tension clasps make putting on nappies a breeze (except for the folding). Be careful though: if they come undone they can scratch you or the baby, which is why some hospitals don't recommend them. We just can't seem to win! At some hospitals they teach a method of wrapping and tucking nappies so they're firm without the use of clasps or pins. This may work for you until baby becomes more mobile.

You can also buy pre-folded nappies that fasten with velcro, but these are expensive and take longer to dry.

Some women say 'hang the environment', and use nothing but disposables. This is something you must make your own decision about. By the way, even disposables are not foolproof for the uninitiated. I shamefacedly admit to trying to put the first one on sideways and wondering why it didn't seem to fit.

Photographs

By now you probably have lots of photos of either mum or dad with the newborn. But before you leave hospital, make sure someone gets a photo of the whole family together. You'll treasure this one later.

DAY 7

We've finally made our baby's name official (much to the relief of the nurses): Rupert Alexander. Rupert is 'thriving' — he's now heavier than his original birth weight and though he had a blotchy face and neck (a slight bacterial infection treated with antibiotics) it's now cleared up.

Despite a vast improvement, I'm still rather stiff and sore in the nether regions and want to have a bit more rest, and attend a couple of the hospital's postnatal exercise classes (baby's feeding pattern permitting) before I leave. I can't imagine coping with my new charge alone at home, the way I'm feeling physically. So I've decided (after consultation with the obstetrician) to stay on for an extra couple of days. Fortunately the hospital can accommodate me.

The exercise class was at 10.30 a.m. Rupert began his feed at 9.30 a.m., and fortunately finished just in time for me to make a mad sprint to the physiotherapy room (leaving him in the nursery in capable hands). I found that there was a different set of exercises for those who'd had caesareans and those who'd had vaginal births. You could spot the women who'd had vaginal births as they were sitting on inflated rubber cushions to relieve the pain from their episiotomies. The women who'd had caesareans were having trouble sitting down! I felt like an old crock trying to get onto the exercise mat in slow motion, compared with my former spritely self. It made me realise just how much of a shock to the system a caesarean is, and how long it was going to take to fully recover. In fact I worried that my muscles would never regain their former elasticity.

The physiotherapist gave us a list of the exercises, and warned that we must practise on a daily basis in order to get our bodies back into shape. I was glad I'd stayed in hospital long enough to take advantage of these motivating sessions, and made a resolution to stick to the daily exercise routine when home. But then, who keeps resolutions ...!

Exercise tips

Your hospital may offer daily physiotherapy classes to help get you back into shape. *Go to them!* There will be many great excuses to avoid this (you're feeding the baby, you're exhausted and need a nap) but weeks or months later, when you view your sagging tummy with despair, you'll be sorry you didn't put in the effort!

Try doing some extra tummy work while lying on your firm hospital bed. Even just a couple of minutes a day will help. Remember, if you can't spare the time to shape up when your every need is being tended to, there's probably little chance you'll be motivated to stick to a routine when you get home. It's a bore, but remember those pelvic floor exercises which are so important for bladder control. You wouldn't want to put up with incontinence as well!

Dining out

While you're still in hospital, take the opportunity (if it's offered or allowed) to go out for dinner with your partner, leaving baby with the night nurse. This is a wonderful treat, one which you probably won't savour again for some time; nevertheless, be prepared to feel like you're missing a limb. The first separation from baby can be hard to bear — a tugging of the heartstrings you couldn't begin to imagine before the event. You may be over-emotional so take some tissues, just in case. (And don't forget a soft cushion to sit on if you have stitches!)

DAY 8

This being my last night in hospital we had organised a very special treat: the nurses were to look after Rupert while Tristan and I went out to dinner. I could hardly wait.

There's a good Italian restaurant right across the road from the hospital. I dressed carefully in an outfit I had packed especially for the occasion, and put on proper make-up for the first time. Then we wheeled Rupert, who was fast asleep, to the nursery, and made sure the nurses had our phone number. Thank goodness the restaurant was so close — we can hardly bear to let him out of our sight!

We had a lovely romantic evening, and toasted our family's future with a bottle of chilled white (I sipped moderately, aware of baby's breastmilk). What a feeling of freedom — just the two of us, having an intimate chat over a leisurely candle-lit meal. Mind you, we were looking forward to seeing our son again by the time dinner ended. We missed the plaintive 'waaah'. And there was no way we were going to leave our valuable charge in someone else's keep for too long. He's so new and precious, we felt we had to be constantly there, guarding him.

Goodness, if we worry while he's in a hospital nursery surrounded by qualified staff, and us only metres away, how are we going to be when we engage our first baby-sitter!

Looking ahead

- Call your local baby clinic, referred to from now on as child health centre (they have different names in each state), and arrange to see them within 2 weeks of arriving home. It's good to make contact before any problems arise, and get to know the nurses, so you'll feel comfortable calling for help. Remember, you may have to wait a while before you can get an appointment.
- If you can't cope with breastfeeding by the time you leave hospital, you could book in for a few days at a private hospital which offers postnatal care.
- Or ask the hospital's lactation specialist if you can come back to her for advice.
- Or pay an early visit to your child health centre (the nurses there are often lactation consultants as well).
- Or arrange for a lactation consultant to visit you at home (home-nursing visits by registered nurses are usually covered by private medical insurance).
- Or ask your child health centre for a referral to a family care cottage, and spend a day under the supervision of child health nurses.
- Consider organising a nappy wash service, at least for the first month, if you haven't already. You'll have more than enough to cope with when you get home without loads of dirty nappies as well.
- Streams of well wishers to the house may also be more than you can cope with. You're going to need plenty of rest (and get very little). Seriously consider banning visitors until you're sure you feel up to it, or at least give them instructions as to when not to call (say between noon and 3 p.m.). And certainly ban house guests, unless it's someone very close who you really want around to help.

- If parents or friends have offered assistance, ask them to cook you some meals which you can put in the freezer. A meal which can be microwaved in minutes will prove invaluable. Or request help with household chores, like washing, cleaning and ironing.

- If you've no help, arrange a weekly or fortnightly cleaning service if you can afford it.

- Consider your telephone needs: an answering machine so you can feed or sleep undisturbed; or a portable phone, which you can put beside you when you're feeding, for those who like to gossip.

- Get dimmers attached to the main light in your bedroom, or wherever you breastfeed at night.

- Don't make any plans to renovate, or move house, during the first 6 months.

A father's view

Taking time off work
Try to arrange a few days off when the baby is born. This is such a marvellous and inspirational time, you will want to savour every second. Most employers are more than happy to see you enjoy it to the full (just like they did when they had their child) but remember to make arrangements in advance.

Some fathers prefer to take time off once mother and child arrive back home. It may mean that you have to juggle hours off work during the first week, but it allows you to spend a week or two at home with your new family.

Controlling the visitors
You might like to take charge of the stream of visitors and keep them down to a manageable flow, for baby and mother, rather than launch a full-scale social event. Do try and get visitors to observe the visiting hours — it will make it easier for everyone.

Breaking the news
The natural temptation will be to ring every person in your contact book but beware, this can have disastrous consequences — you might have 20 people descend on you at once. It's far better to ring selectively, and in stages depending on importance, to stagger the visits so that they fit in with you. But don't delay or she won't have any visitors at all, and then you'll really be in trouble!

Don't forget the vases
Within hours of the birth, the visitors — and flowers — will start to flow in. Birth centres and maternity wards do a sterling job, but you may need extra vases to cope with what appears to be the contents of a large florist shop. If so, bring in all the (older) vases and containers you can find, packing them carefully. Now all you have to do is remember to take them home.

And yes, you can bring her flowers each time (even if you do visit more than once a day!).

Home can be a lonely place

It is very hard for a new father to leave a little piece of domestic bliss and return to an empty house. Leaving the hospital is a bit like walking out of a movie theatre — all action, emotion and intensity inside; and outside, another world — utterly different and a bit lonely. Only the promise of the next visit to see 'the family' stops any feeling of melancholy. Mind you, by the time you begin to get used to it, the baby will be home and it all changes again.

For some of the time being home alone is an opportunity to do 'your thing', but this can soon lose its appeal. Some of us will rapidly come to appreciate just how much our partner does by way of washing, ironing, tidying and paying bills. And she's going to do it all with a baby as well?

Survival techniques

Make sure you have enough food to eat and know how to do a load of washing. For the next couple of days you're on your own. Stock up the week before on essential and easy-to-prepare supplies. Remember, you may not get home from the hospital until after 10 p.m. You'll be surprised at how easy it is to forget about food when you are having so much fun with your family. You will become an instant expert on take-away options and the finer points of making that great lifesaver — two-minute noodles. Try to avoid having to resort (as I did) to a diet of toasted Vegemite sandwiches made from last week's crusts.

A word on names

Because hospitals are terribly efficient places, and everything has a name (and a tidy place), it will be assumed that your child has one too. Naming a child is truly a special and significant event. You may, like some parents, wish to see what your child looks like before deciding on Harold Horatio Horace III (not a great name for a girl). The nursing staff may well give you disapproving looks as you gaze down upon baby 'Blank', but don't be pressured. Take your time.

Holding your baby correctly takes practice

The first time you hold your child is a memorable moment. But you'll find no instruction booklets, or illustrations on the outside of the packaging! Mothers learn to manage it and with a bit of practice you will master it too. Your baby will look so fragile and delicate, but with a little care you can't really go wrong. First, establish eye contact and gently lift your child, making sure to keep the head supported at all times. This is usually best done in the crook of your arm. Bring the baby up and close to your chest ... Well, you know the rest — start making strange cooing noises and grin from ear to ear.

Baby blues — you can survive them too

Baby blues is such a delightful term for your partner turning into a howling blob of jelly just because you said 'Hello, how was your day?' Don't even bother asking 'What did I say?'! Plunging hormone levels act like a powerful drug, and can turn that happy smiling person you love so much into a complete wreck in seconds. There is only one remedy: support and patience. Don't feel victimised or react in kind. Just go with the flow, stay calm and let her pour it all out.

Fitting the baby capsule or restraint

If you haven't already done so a week in advance (as your partner instructed), now is the time to get a qualified installer to fit the capsule or 0–4 years car seat. This is a vital piece of safety equipment so if anything is unclear, go back to the supplier or installer and let them demonstrate. Fitting it yourself 'because men know about these things' may not be enough. Note that some cars are not rated for certain restraints and it is worthwhile calling the manufacturer or motoring organisation to find out the facts. Remember, you are dealing with a foreign object, not something straightforward like a reciprocating engine. You'll know it's a whole new ball game because you can't get your hands dirty.

Breasts

You will probably notice that your partner's breasts grow significantly when the milk comes in — but they're not for you! The best thing you can do during the next few days is find a fruit shop that sells organic cabbages and buy a packet of frozen peas for when she gets home — and no, you can't eat those either.

Sending out 'thank-you' cards

I know this sounds ridiculous, but it took us 9 weeks to thank the generous people who came to the hospital with good wishes, champagne and flowers. (If I come and visit you and am not thanked for 3 months, I won't take offence.) You could try to do some thank-you notes while you are alone at home, or at the hospital.

1 WEEK OLD

MILESTONES
- Sucks efficiently.
- Demonstrates difference in pitch when crying.

WHAT THEY NEVER TELL YOU THIS WEEK

- Caring for your baby in a hospital or birthing centre is one thing; caring for him when you get home can come as a big shock so be prepared.

- It's quite normal for your baby to have one unsettled period per day — usually in the afternoon or early evening — and one unsettled day per week.

- Overtiredness is a common cause of crying which can be prevented.

- It's best to always sleep baby in his own bed, in the same room (away from the activity of the house), so he learns to distinguish sleep time from play time.

- You'll have emotional and physical ups and downs, the euphoria of having your baby competing with the round-the-clock demands of your new job.

- You'll have very little sleep, and be exhausted like never before.

- You may feel insecure, even panic stricken, by your new responsibilities.

- You may feel timid about venturing outside with the baby.

- You may be concerned about bleeding, discomfort, or using the toilet.

- You may have night sweats because of hormonal imbalance.

- You may not have time to prepare proper meals, or tidy up the house.

- Visitors may be the last thing you want.

- If you allow your breasts to become hard and swollen, you risk developing mastitis.

- *All this is perfectly normal.*

THINGS TO DO THIS WEEK

- Register baby's name (if you haven't already).

- Have baby's name added to your Medicare card.

CHAPTER TWO
---

1 week old

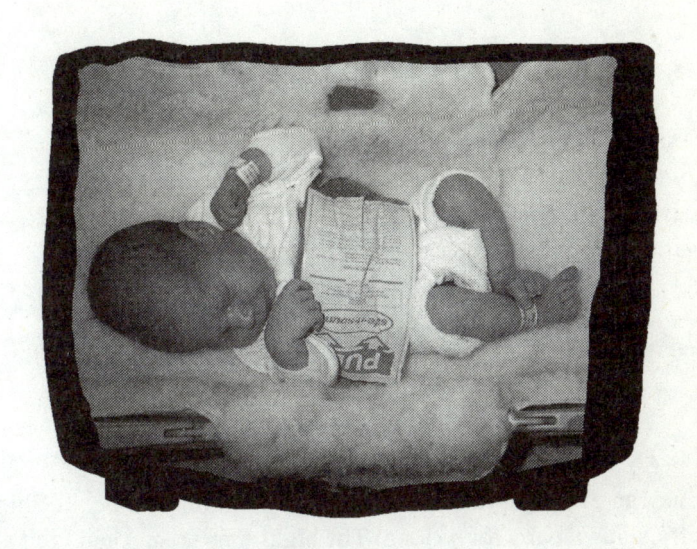

DAY 8

After fond farewells to hospital staff, and many last-minute photos, we gingerly carried the baby in his capsule downstairs into the crisp winter sunshine. It was such a thrill, taking our baby home. Everything looked wondrous and fresh after the confines of the hospital. A whole new world awaited us.

I felt excited, like a newlywed, as we sailed through the sparkling city, savouring the glimpses of bright blue harbour.

Ten minutes later we were crossing the threshold. Rupert was still sleeping, so we gently transferred him to his new cradle in the corner of our bedroom, and stood back to admire our achievement. We had chilled our prized bottle of expensive French champagne, the one we were too tired to drink after the birth. Now was the perfect moment to break it open.

> *Later that afternoon I walked into our bedroom and was momentarily stunned to find myself confronted with the cradle, and a living, breathing creature inside. It was as if I'd had a memory lapse, had forgotten that we now have a baby, and our life has irrevocably changed.*

Your baby this week

Baby still has no strength in his neck to support his head. His movements may be a little jerky. He will cry a lot — after all, this is his only form of communication. If you are lucky, he will also spend a great deal of time sleeping — newborns average 14–18 hours sleep over 24 hours. Visually, he'll be more aware of contrast (black and white) than colour, for the first 6 weeks.

The ecstasy

No-one can ever tell you how wonderful it's going to be. To think I put off having a baby for so long! The highs that Tristan and I felt after the birth were matched only by the ecstasy of our wedding day, yet the feelings continued, and intensified, hour after hour. Suddenly, our life had a new dimension, a source of constant joy and fulfilment. This was a bond I had never realised was possible, especially for someone who never claimed to be 'maternal'. And a sense of sharing with my husband, like two cats wallowing in the cream. It's good to keep this picture in mind as you wade through the troughs that inevitably follow.

The agony

They never tell you how hard it's going to be! Although the first week at home may pass in a blissful trance — particularly if you have family or friends who are bringing you food, helping out around the house, and taking turns to hold the baby — it will soon dawn on you that coping with the demands of such a wee little thing can prove an unexpectedly huge drain on your time and energy. It is difficult to explain to anyone who hasn't been through it just where all that time goes!

For the next few weeks, your life will revolve around the feeding and sleeping habits of your baby. In between, there are snatches of time for bathing the baby, changing nappies, soothing the baby, changing soiled clothes (yours and his), washing and drying nappies, bunny rugs and clothing, getting yourself dressed and fed and, if you're lucky, managing to cook a meal, do some housework or take a quick nap.

On top of all that is the lack of sleep. You may have to manage on just a couple of hours some nights. And there's the insecurity of this being unexplored territory. Am I doing it right? Is he crying too much? Feeding enough?

Under such stress, even the most complacent of us will become frazzled at times, and relationships are likely to be strained. It's okay, as long as you both understand that this is normal, since your life is undergoing such a major upheaval.

Bear in mind that things will improve after the first 6 to 12 weeks, when you're more confident and competent, and the baby starts settling into a routine. Hang in until then.

Get some rest

You'll always find things to do during the day which are 'more important' than resting, but try to make resting (and eating) a priority. Take the phone off the hook and dive for the bed the moment he goes down after the lunchtime feed. Don't try to fit in a quick chore first — you don't know how long his sleep will last. At the very least, put your feet up with a cup of tea for 10 minutes — you deserve it! If it helps you relax, ask a friend or relative to baby-sit in the other room while you take a nap (maybe they could fold some clothes as well). At this stage, it's better to have the house a mess than have you run down. You'll cope much better with the baby if you look after yourself as well.

> ## Take a break
>
> - Pluck up the courage to venture out into the big wide world with baby.
> - Walk the pram around the block, or put the baby in a sling and go for a stroll (a good way to get him to sleep).
> - Take the baby and visit a friend (who has children) for coffee.
> - Ask a parent or friend to look after the baby for half an hour, while you go out for a coffee or a walk.

DAY 10

2 a.m. Switch on the bed-lamp in response to the 'waaah, waaah' cry. Reach into the cradle by the bed. Prop myself up on pillows, half asleep, and put baby to breast, mumbling to myself 'Which breast did I start with last time? Must offer him the other one. Should I change his nappy before or after?'. Tristan was good enough to rouse himself and chat to me throughout the procedure (a novelty which would soon wear off!). It was 6.15 a.m. before I settled the baby back to sleep, almost time for Tristan to get up on a normal working day.

You don't realise that although the actual breastfeeding may take only 30 to 40 minutes, the period is extended by the burping in between breasts, then the final burping, nappy changing and settling afterwards. For a novice like me, with a baby who possets, that's about $1\frac{1}{2}$ hours snatched from your night every time you feed, although I'm told feeds do get faster as you become more practised.

At 11.30 a.m. we realised that we hadn't yet had breakfast and were both still in our dressing gowns. We had to giggle at each other. This baby business was a lot more hectic than we'd thought!

Posseting

To 'posset' is to bring up milk after a feed. It's annoying because it's messy, and worrying because you wonder whether the baby's getting enough nourishment. However, it's quite common due to baby's underdeveloped digestive system, and no cause for concern if he's still alert, happy and gaining weight. Some babies hardly posset at all while others posset so much that their parents are rarely seen without a nappy or bunny rug draped over their shoulders to protect their clothing!
(See also Posseting or reflux, pages 168–71.)

Sleeping arrangements

Many mothers prefer to sleep the baby in a cradle in the main bedroom, at least for the first few weeks. There are others who can't sleep when baby is in the room because of constant snuffles or whimpers, and opt for the nursery or sibling's room.

Whatever you choose, child health nurses advise consistency from the very beginning, always settling baby to sleep in the same room, in his own bed (bassinet or cot), away from the activity of the house. As well as giving a sense of security, this helps him understand that sleep time is distinct from play time. You may think that a newborn wouldn't know the difference, but the nurses assure me it's worth getting into the routine from birth.

Some mothers favour settling baby in a pram which can be rocked and wheeled from room to room as you're working. But apart from the lack of a consistent 'home base', health authorities strongly warn against sleeping babies in prams which convert to strollers. There have been cases in Australia where babies have slipped through the gap at the end and have been strangled or suffocated.

Tristan and I wanted the baby in our room. Baby monitor or not, it's reassuring to be close to baby during the night, so you can check his sleeping position and be aware of any sounds. And if you position the cradle close to your bed you'll be able to scoop the baby up to breastfeed, or pop in a dummy or rock him to sleep without even leaving your bed.

A recent New Zealand study into cot death claims statistics show that sleeping infants in the same bedroom as their parents at night will reduce the risk of Sudden Infant Death Syndrome (SIDS) — although they don't know exactly why. However, at the time of writing, Australian SIDS groups feel the evidence is not sufficiently convincing to include in their recommendations.

Some parents like to sleep with the baby, but sharing a bed is not recommended by the experts as baby might become too hot, risk suffocation due to soft bedding or pillows, or risk being rolled upon. Pillows placed vertically each side of the baby as bolsters may also cause overheating.

It's a good idea to get a dimmer attached to the bedroom or nursery light and leave it on low all night, or buy a toddler's nightlight for a soft glow. You don't want to stimulate baby (or yourself) with bright lights at feed time.

Minimising risk of cot death

Most cases of SIDS occur during the first 6 months. The following guidelines are suggested by the National SIDS Council of Australia in their publication *Reducing the Risk of SIDS*:

- Sleep baby on the back.
- Keep your baby in a smoke-free environment during pregnancy and for at least the first year after birth.
- Do not let your baby become too hot.
- Breastfeed your baby, if possible.
- Use layers of light bedding. Doonas, thick quilts, cot bumpers and soft toys in the cot are not recommended.
- Use a firm, clean, well-fitting mattress and no pillow.
- Don't put baby on water beds or beanbags.
- Put baby's feet at the bottom of the cot. (This is to stop baby wriggling down under the bed covers.)

Cradles, cots and bassinets

It helps to have a cradle or bassinet you can jiggle, either from side to side or end to end. Rapid rhythmic jiggling (as against slow rocking) can be an amazingly effective way to get the baby to sleep, even though you'd think it would have the opposite effect! My favourite style is the old-fashioned wicker bassinet on a stand. They're stable, yet light enough to jiggle, and the bassinet part can be carried from room to room when baby's awake, so he can watch you while you work. Beware of rocking cradles that can lock at an angle, tipping the baby onto his stomach and causing suffocation. For safety's sake, rocking cradles should always be secured in a non-rocking position when baby is left alone.

It's fine to use a cot right from the start if you prefer (maybe one is just being vacated by an older brother or sister), although it does seem rather a vast area for a newborn. Some mothers make it cosier by inserting a 'snuggle bed' (a shaped tea-tree mattress with firm base), but this practice was at time of writing being investigated by SIDS as a possible risk factor, along with tri-pillows, or boomerang pillows. This is because of the risks of overheating, and the possibility of baby turning his head into the soft material and suffocating. Bolsters and wedges around the inside of cots are not recommended either, as they may cause overheating, poor air circulation or accidental suffocation.

It's important not to overheat baby by piling on too many blankets, or using a thick doona. In cold weather, it's better to dress baby warmly, with singlet, socks and overgarments, and add as many layers as necessary. (Loose-weave cotton blankets, like the ones most hospitals use, are a safe bet.) You can test whether baby is too hot by placing your hand on his chest or back, to see if he's sweaty. He should feel comfortably warm, but not moist.

A woollen underblanket, or even a lambswool placed under the sheet, will make the bed cosier, as well as protecting the mattress against any accidental leakage.

Pillows shouldn't be used, but if baby possets frequently, cover the head area of the sheet with something absorbent, such as a cloth nappy. Then cover this with an empty pillowcase, bunny rug or folded sheet, so it's smooth against his delicate skin.

When decorating the cradle or cot with bells, baubles and mobiles, keep in mind that baby can only focus up to 20–30 cm at this stage, so hang objects fairly close. Be careful, though, of cords, necklaces, bonnets with ribbons and toys which can wrap around baby's neck or limbs. Musical wind-up mobiles, which play lullaby songs, are great soothers and will become an endless source of fascination as baby moves through various stages of awareness and development.

Black-and-white visuals

During these first weeks, baby is attracted to contrast rather than colour. Using some black-and-white items in his environment will help baby focus his eyes.

- Cut out shapes from cardboard or paper.
- Hang some black-and-white smiling faces (easily made from white card or paper).
- Buy a black-and-white cloth book.
- Find a black-and-white soccer ball.
- Seek out *101 Dalmatians*-inspired toys.
- Wear a black-and-white T-shirt.

Night duty

The choice of who stays awake at night feeding times is an individual one, obviously made to suit your lifestyle and temperaments. Usually it's the mother's responsibility, although sometimes male partners will enthusiastically stay awake with you (at least for the first few nights) to share the experience. Others feel it's important to keep one of the team alert and refreshed for the working day ahead, and spare the father as much as possible, even to the extent of breastfeeding and sleeping the remainder of the night in the spare room if the partner's a light sleeper. From my research and experience, though, most men quickly learn to sleep through an earthquake!

Because you'll be so tired, consider letting your partner take over one of the night feeds every so often. This is easier if you're bottle-feeding, of course, but breastfeeding mothers can always express enough milk for a bottle. That's if your full breasts and mothering instincts will allow you to sleep through!

Night feeding tips

- Aim to keep baby's waking time to a minimum. With practice you should be able to feed and settle within half an hour, rather than an hour or more.

- Keep the lighting as dim as possible.

- If baby needs changing, do it before the feed, not after (even though after may seem biologically most logical), to avoid any disruption just before resettling.

- Consider using a disposable nappy, a nappy liner, or two cloth nappies if necessary, so baby doesn't have to be changed during the night (unless the nappy is dirty, or baby is prone to nappy rash). He will settle back to sleep faster if not disturbed and the benefits of baby and mother having more sleep usually outweigh the disadvantages of a wet nappy.

- Try breastfeeding lying on your side in bed, with baby alongside you. It doesn't suit everyone, but could work for you. Just make sure you don't fall asleep and roll onto the baby.

- Get into the habit of communicating with baby as little as possible during night feeds. As he becomes older, any talking and smiling will only stimulate him, and keep him awake longer.

Sleeping and feeding schedule

Most experts agree that newborns should be fed on demand, at intervals of between 2 and 5 hours, depending on their size and appetite. Hopefully in a few weeks your baby will settle into a pattern, feeding every 4 hours or so, with a nap in between. This gives you much more freedom to plan your day, as well as a reasonable space between feeds. But obviously babies don't function like clockwork, so don't be concerned if feeding intervals vary. And be warned — just as you feel you're set in a comfortable routine, babies are apt to do a complete turnaround, just to jolt you out of your complacency and show they're still boss.

In an ideal world, your baby will sleep up to 18 hours a day (sounds too good to be true, doesn't it). What they don't tell you, is that on some occasions the baby may cry right through his usual sleep time. And then be overtired and cry some more. In fact, it's quite normal for a baby to have at least one unsettled period per day (usually in the afternoon or early evening) and at least one unsettled day per week. Some babies can be unsettled for the whole day or night for the first few weeks. Unfortunately no-one ever tells you this either, so you're liable to make matters worse by blaming yourself, rather than accepting it as normal and taking it in your stride. (See also Basic settling techniques, pages 95–6 and Ideal routine, pages 113–14.)

Expectations versus reality

Just as baby can turn from sweet angel to red wizened crying ball in a matter of seconds, so your day can change from good to ghastly, and back again, without warning. Be prepared to cope with the unpredictable. The first few weeks are crazy because at this stage there is no pattern. It's just a matter of responding to your baby's constant needs — now! And it takes time to learn how to correctly interpret those needs.

Forget those rosy images of motherhood you saw in the magazines and in movies — the ones that make you feel by comparison that there's something wrong with you. The serene, smiling, well-groomed mum, nursing the equally serene, prettily dressed, cherubic baby, is a rare find indeed. It's actually quite normal for a new mother to be stressed, cross or upset. When having a first baby, your expectations and reality rarely coincide.

Most of us probably thought that babies were generally fairly quiet, docile things, who went to sleep naturally, and slept most of the time. We didn't realise that crying was the norm, and going to sleep was a technique that had to be learned! Most of us thought that going out with a little baby would be easy, not a massive undertaking often hardly worth the effort! Mind you, I have seen 'dream babies' at other people's homes but I'm sure they're in the minority.

Looking back at my diary, my husband and I seemed incredibly disorganised and out of control during the first few months. At the time, it seemed unavoidable; but in hindsight, I feel we would have benefited from some good practical advice on organisation.

Getting organised

- Try to split the duties more methodically between partners when you're both at home, rather than attempt to share the load together. Allocate one person to 'baby' duties and the other to 'home/self' duties (like cleaning and eating), then swap. You may not see as much of each other, or have the same feeling of companionship, but at least more things will get done.

- Allocate specific chores to your partner, and communicate how important it is for you to receive this help without having to nag.

- Use mornings to do necessary household chores, such as putting out the washing or deciding what's for dinner, as afternoons can deteriorate rapidly.

- When and if you find the time to prepare a casserole or soup, always make a large quantity and freeze some for another meal. And if family members offer to cook and freeze meals for you, accept without hesitation! There will be nights you'll be so exhausted that a pre-prepared meal, which can be microwaved in minutes, will mean nourishment — rather than collapsing into bed without any dinner at all.

- Keep two buckets full of nappy wash solution — one for the nappies, and one to soak baby's clothes until you're ready for a wash. They'll end up much cleaner.
- Stack all cloth nappies pre-folded so they're ready to put on.
- Try storing complete outfits, folded or rolled up together — jumpsuit, singlet, socks, pilcher, nappy — so you can grab a bundle in a hurry (or when the room is dark) and know you have everything.
- Always have the baby bag packed with all the necessities. Make a list of the items you're likely to need (including sorbolene or nappy wipes for changing in case water is unavailable, bibs, sunhat) so you can check them off as you pack.
- If breastfeeding, think about what you wear when you go out. It's so easy and acceptable to breastfeed in public, and you may avoid having an excursion cut short because of a hungry or unsettled baby.

DAY 11

Optimistically, we decided to go shopping for supplies. Our first big venture out. Rupert looked so tiny in his blue pram as we wheeled him proudly up and down the aisles. People would stop and peer in, and marvel at his size. I've never spoken to so many strangers in a supermarket before! Fortunately, he slept through the whole expedition without a peep.

By the time we got home I was rather tired and sore. Maybe I was overdoing it. After all, they had told me to get lots of rest in the first week. But we were in for a rude surprise — a gruelling 8-hour stretch of crying, screaming and more crying that went down in history as our 'black afternoon'.

I fed at 4 p.m., thinking he'd be settled by about 5.30 p.m., as usual. At 5.45 p.m. I tiptoed gratefully out of the bedroom and collapsed into an armchair. 'Waaah!' came the sound 5 minutes later. We spent the next hour frantically trying to quieten him, until it was time for his next feed. Surely he'd go down after that! Same thing — settle, but false alarm. And so it went on.

I can't explain what a state we were in by mid-evening, or why it was so tortuous. There's just something about the sound of your baby's constant crying, the way it grates on your nerves, tugs at your soul, your frustration at not knowing why the poor little thing's so upset, your total inability to do anything about it. Tristan and I started snapping at each other, which didn't improve things, but unfortunately seems to come with the territory.

Finally, at midnight, he settled. We hadn't had any dinner, but who cared. We collapsed into bed, and were rewarded with an unbroken 8 hours sleep. The baby was obviously exhausted too.

Overtiredness

No-one tells you that one of the most common causes of crying is overtiredness. You may put your baby's whingeing down to boredom, wind, colic or unhappiness, when what he needs is a good sleep.

It's important to put baby to bed as soon as he starts to get tired, but in order to do this, you must learn to recognise the signs in your baby — and these are not necessarily the signs we usually associate with being tired, like yawning and blinking.

It may be that our valiant efforts to soothe (walking with the baby, singing, or rocking) are in fact prolonging the crying — by stimulating the baby and keeping him awake when all the poor thing wants to do is sleep. Soothe him with hushing sounds and stroke his head or tummy, or leave him for a little while to cry himself to sleep. It may be hard for you to do, but an overtired baby will fall asleep faster this way than if he is continually picked up and stimulated by attempts to pacify him.

If your baby does not cry, yet stays awake when it's sleep time, simply put him down and let him be. In some cases, waiting for him to display the signs of tiredness means you'll have waited too long. Make an effort to get him into the habit of sleeping, as sleep breeds sleep!

> **Common signs of tiredness**
> - grizzling
> - jerky movements
> - hand clenching
> - frowning
> - facial grimacing

Colic

I was always uncertain what this was, while my husband thought it was something horses got. Other people used the tag with gay abandon, but to me it was a mysterious word, which everyone seemed to interpret vaguely, applying it to any baby under the age of 3 or 4 months who cried a great deal.

In fact, the word is derived from the Latin and Greek for 'pertaining to the colon' and, according to the *Macquarie Dictionary*, it refers to 'paroxysmal pain in the abdomen or bowels'. So it would appear to be a condition related to wind. However, it's loosely used by experts and mothers alike to refer to babies who cry long and often without explanation, or who cry for various reasons ranging from hunger and heartburn to overtiredness and tension. (The term 'reflux' is also used loosely in similar fashion.)

There are a few different medications available from the pharmacy for colic, but they are specifically designed to help bring up wind — so are useless if wind is not in fact the cause of the crying.

The silly thing is that paediatricians can't even agree on whether colic exists. I must say, it would help to have an accepted definition of the condition before trying to prove its existence. The most sensible definition I've heard comes from a health professional with a sense of humour: 'Colic stands for Cause Obscure Lengthy Infant Crying.'

Obviously there are babies who cry chronically, often in the late afternoon or evening, and who refuse to be consoled, and it is extremely distressing for parents. The only good news is that this sort of behaviour usually stops at around 3 months.

If this is colic, so be it. But if someone says you have a colicky baby, ask them to be more specific!

More crying tips

If baby is not crying because he's hungry, hot, cold, wet or in pain, it may simply be because he is feeling insecure, or just needs help to get to sleep. As well as the standard settling techniques (see pages 95–6), here are some other options:

- Curl up with baby tummy to tummy in a warm bed, with the room darkened and quiet, and maximum skin to skin contact (a good position to breastfeed as well).
- Try a deep warm bath, and some baby massage.
- Rock with baby in a chair, and sing or play music.
- Walk rhythmically with baby over the shoulder (ancient tribal remedy).
- Put baby in a pouch. That way he can be close to you and soothed by your warmth and movement, while you get on with other tasks.
- A baby hammock can be wonderful to help settle, or give you a break. Babies love them, but don't leave them in the hammock for long periods (an hour at the very most).

DAY 12

We woke to find the house an absolute mess from the day before. The baby wanted immediate attention: we were plunged into the raging whirlpool again. This was life out of control — no time for breakfast, no time to clean up. We tore around, rinsing out clothes that had been posseted on, changing (us and/or him), dealing with wet and dirty nappies, fetching clean towels to throw over our shoulder (to catch the possets), walking the floor, feeding, burping, patting, rocking, singing, arguing, crying. It's hard to explain how two people can spend a whole day at home running around after the baby, and do nothing else. How can someone so small dictate our lives?

Tristan cooked us some fish for dinner. Bad timing. We ate it, cold, some 3 hours later. Delicious!

If you're breastfeeding

What no-one ever tells you is that although breastfeeding is so often depicted as a blissful spell of serenity and oneness with your baby (which indeed it can be), it is not like that for everyone. Some new mothers find it a daunting, frustrating or painful task.

You may well have the expectation that feeding is a relatively simple and automatic procedure, over with in 20–30 minutes.

However, depending on your milk, and the baby's sucking and burping habits, the breastfeeding itself can take anything from 20 minutes (10 minutes on each breast) to an hour (yes, 30 minutes on each!). But add extra time (maybe 15 minutes) for the burping (and sometimes snoozing or playing) between each breast and after the feed, and in some cases the bringing up of milk and trying again. Then, of course, you have to change nappies and settle the baby down to sleep. So the whole procedure can take as long as $1\frac{1}{2}$ hours (at least in the beginning, while you and the baby are still learners).

This means that if you have an unsettled baby who feeds twice during the night (say midnight and 4 a.m.), or a baby who demands more frequent feeds, you could have a total of about 3 hours snatched from your sleeping time each night; then, of course, you're up again for the breakfast feed and the start of a new day. No wonder you're tired!

Feeding on demand

The modern catchcry is 'feed on demand, not by the clock'. But don't take this too literally and run yourself into the ground. Some mothers interpret demand feeding to mean 'feed the baby every time he cries', but crying doesn't necessarily mean baby is hungry. Feed on demand, within reason.

Some small babies may need 2-hourly feeds for the first 6 weeks until the milk supply becomes established and their small tummies can hold more milk. But after that intervals of between 3 to 5 hours are more usual, as long as baby is gaining weight. The Nursing Mothers' Association recommends at least 6 feeds in 24 hours for the first 3 months.

Breastfeeding tips

- Breastfeed on demand (usually every 3 to 5 hours, depending on baby's size and appetite).
- Put on the answering machine or take the phone off the hook. Alternatively, keep the phone by your chair (with the ringer volume turned down low), as someone's sure to call! This is where a portable, rather than a mobile, phone can come in handy.
- Sit well back in the chair. Try resting your feet on a small stool or two telephone books, to help keep your back straight and knees up.
- Have pillows under your arm and/or on your lap to rest baby on, and behind your neck if necessary.
- Experiment with different positions. Try holding baby with left arm and cupping left breast with right hand or try supporting baby with right arm (hand cupping his head) and holding left breast with left hand, or hold baby under arm (football hold), draining milk from the underarm side.
- Take a deep breath and relax your body before baby latches on.
- It's okay to stay on one breast for 20–30 minutes, until it is empty or baby finishes — emptying the breast helps avoid mastitis, and ensures he gets a good balance of foremilk and hindmilk. (As he gets older, and more efficient at sucking, it will take less time.)
- Get into the habit of always offering the second breast — even if baby doesn't take it this time, he may do so at another feed.
- Mark your bra with a safety pin (or other indicator) to show which breast you started with this time, so you can alternate at each feed.
- Have a glass of water at your side when you feed. It's normal to become thirsty or hungry when so much high-quality fluid is leaving your body.

- Some babies need a 'comfort suck' in order to settle. Often this urge can be mistaken for hunger. A baby with a need to suck is best put back on the first breast, so that he can suck without being hit with a surge of milk he doesn't want. You may choose to use a dummy instead.

Cracked or bleeding nipples

I've known women whose nipples bled throughout the first 5 or 6 weeks. It's worth mentioning that a friend of mine nearly fainted with fright when her baby vomited up what seemed a huge amount of blood after feeding. Thinking it was an internal haemorrhage, she rushed him to the doctor, only to find that this was the baby's efficient digestive system at work, accepting the breastmilk but rejecting the blood that came with it!

If your nipples are sore, don't feel you're doomed to put up with it. Seek professional help urgently, and have someone check that you are positioning the baby correctly. In some cases, this is all that is needed to solve the problem.

As a preventative measure, do your best to keep your nipples dry. This is almost impossible when you're breastfeeding, as your breasts will leak after a feed. But it helps to avoid using anything synthetic against your nipples, like plastic-lined pads or polyester bras. Use cotton only. Remember to rub some breastmilk onto the nipples to help the healing process. And expose your nipples to air for about 15 minutes after feeding if you can.

Some women who are troubled by extremely sore or cracked nipples, but don't wish to turn to formula, use a breast pump as an interim measure, and feed baby expressed milk in a bottle or cup.

Soft silicone nipple shields with tiny holes (also used for women with flat or inverted nipples) may enable you to continue breastfeeding, by reducing the pain and helping prevent further cracking and irritation from baby's sucking. These are a lifesaver for some women who would otherwise have to resort to expressing milk to feed their baby, or switch to formula. But, unfortunately, not all women report success. Some say they don't stop the pain, some find them too awkward to use, and some babies (especially those older than 3 weeks) won't accept them.

Experts warn that shields may irritate and cause further damage to nipples, and reduce supply if used long-term as sucking through a shield doesn't stimulate breasts to the same extent. They advise women to use them only as a short-term measure, and only under the guidance of a midwife or lactation consultant.

Tips for engorged breasts

- Hot face-washers, or hot cloth nappies, before a feed and before expressing.
- Hot showers and massage.
- Massage with oil.
- Cold cabbage leaves inside your bra.
- Cold packs (or packets of frozen peas) wrapped in towels.
- Cold face washers (wring out, chill in freezer in plastic bag).
- Breastfeed as much as you can to drain the breasts.
- Empty one swollen breast at each feed if possible.
- Express a little before the feed, and after if necessary.
- If breasts become painful or develop hard lumps or red patches, seek medical advice. This could be the first sign of mastitis.
- Remember, heat before a feed, cold after. (Heat helps the milk flow, cold relieves the pain.)

Mastitis

Mastitis is inflammation of the breast tissue, characterised by engorgement, soreness, hard lumps, a red patch on the skin and flu-like symptoms such as tiredness, headache, chills or a raised temperature. It can occur out of the blue if you miss a feed (for example, if baby sleeps for a 7- or 8-hour stretch), if baby is given a bottle for one feed and you don't express to compensate, or if your breasts are not being emptied sufficiently due to poor attachment. There is usually an accompanying infection, which may be caused by a blocked duct, or may enter the duct via a cracked nipple.

If not treated immediately, mastitis can become more serious and develop into an abscess. See your GP or child health nurse as soon as you notice any of these symptoms. They will probably recommend bedrest, plenty of fluids, warm compresses and long hot showers to get the milk flowing, and massaging the breasts with oil to help express. Cold packs and cabbage leaves help relieve the pain and swelling. You may need antibiotics if the breast is infected (about 50 per cent of cases), although there is a slight risk these could cause rashes, diarrhoea and thrush in the baby.

It's worth noting that natural therapies may be effective. A friend of mine had recurring mastitis, and endured at least 5 separate courses of antibiotics. Finally she visited a naturopath, and was given a herb specifically for mastitis. She never suffered the infection again.

If you have mastitis, it's important to keep feeding regularly in order to empty your breasts, but make sure that baby is properly attached. Massage the red areas or lumps while baby feeds.

Foremilk and hindmilk

While a lot of emphasis used to be placed on the importance of baby getting the right balance of foremilk (the breastmilk that comes out first) and hindmilk (the milk that follows this), most baby care advisors will now tell you not to worry about this. If you always feed baby from one breast, and offer the second, then baby will ensure that he gets the right balance. However it doesn't hurt to be aware of the two milk types.

The foremilk is very watery, thirst quenching and high in protein and sugar. Hindmilk is thicker, and higher in fat and calories — important to satisfy baby, help him settle, and improve weight gain. Feeding for only 5 to 10 minutes at one breast, before changing to the other, could result in an intake of mainly foremilk and an unsatisfied baby. Allowing baby to stay on one breast longer ensures you go beyond the foremilk to the hindmilk (and also ensures you empty the breast, so it refills effectively).

It is useful to keep this difference in mind when expressing milk to store for a later feed. For example, if you habitually express a little milk before feeds, freezing it in stages to build up a bottle, you run the risk of filling a bottle with foremilk only, and it won't be satisfying for baby. It's best to either express for a longer time on one breast, or express both before and at the end of a feed, if possible, to get the hindmilk.

Foods to eat while breastfeeding

In the old days, breastfeeding mothers were advised not to eat strong foods like garlic and onion. But now this is actually seen by some as an advantage, if you want your child to have a sophisticated palate! A recent local study found that breastfed babies whose mothers ate a lot of garlic were more willing than other breastfed babies to eat garlic-flavoured foods when introduced to solids. This could explain why my toddler had cravings for garlic, green olives and capers! The findings also indicated that breastfed babies were quicker to accept solids, and more likely to eat nutritious foods, possibly because of the range of flavours passed on in breastmilk.

That said, you may still be advised to avoid garlic, ginger and spicy foods, such as chilli and satay, because these can upset some babies. Similarly, cabbage, cauliflower, broccoli and brussels sprouts are notorious for causing baby to have wind. You and baby may have no problems, whatever you eat, but it pays to be aware, just in case baby's unsettled periods are sometimes due to the foods you are eating.

Remember, too, that you still need more calcium than normal if you're breastfeeding. That is, you need to eat more than the standard 3 servings of dairy foods or calcium-rich foods per day.

Alcohol and breastfeeding

Expert opinions on the wisdom of imbibing alcohol while breastfeeding vary, and are in some cases contradictory. Some health professionals say a glass of wine or a measure of spirits is fine, and can even help breastfeeding by relaxing the mother (so facilitating let down) and acting as a mild sedative for the baby. Others argue that alcohol can inhibit let down. Some lactation consultants advise not more than one serve of alcohol per day, and then preferably after a feed, to reduce the amount filtering through to the milk. Others suggest that mothers who need a drink a day would be wise to seek counselling, to find out why.

One mother I know chooses to give her baby a bottle of formula instead of a breastfeed if she is going to drink, or if she eats food which she feels might upset the baby. Of course, the amount of time alcohol will remain in the milk (whether it is for one feed or more) depends on the amount consumed. As does the time between taking a drink and the alcohol appearing in the breastmilk (usually a matter of hours, although research in this area is hard to find).

Bear in mind when drinking that if you're over the limit as far as driving goes, then you're over the limit for baby as well. Levels of alcohol in breastmilk are the same as those in your blood, and when breastfeeding it's best to keep well below the danger level.

Burping tips

- Try a gentle circular rub on the back after the feed, while holding him upright or against your shoulder. (You don't need to go into a patting frenzy.)
- Or sit baby up on your knee, with his back straight, and gently rub his tummy.
- Or hold baby in the crook of your arm in a 'c' shape, so his knees are drawn up towards his tummy.
- Or place baby tummy down over your arm, so gentle pressure is exerted on his tummy.
- Try burping in between breasts, or halfway through the bottle, as well as at the end of the feed.
- If there's no burping after 5 minutes, there's no need to persevere.

If you're bottlefeeding

You may feel like an alien at your new mothers' group, forced to defend your position. To make matters worse, it may be hard to find sufficient information on bottlefeeding in all the baby books you've bought. But remember, you probably have valid reasons for not breastfeeding, so don't feel guilty.

Although you miss out on all the advantages breastfeeding has to offer (which I'm sure you've been made well aware of by now), focus on the positives: your baby will still get nutritious food, lots of warmth and love, and, what's more, your partner can be involved in the feeding process, and take an equal share of the load. Maybe one of his jobs could be washing and sterilising at night, making up the day's supply of bottles, or taking over night feeds at the weekend!

When making up the bottles, bear in mind that from now until 3 months, the quantity of milk baby needs per day is generally calculated at 150 ml of milk per kilogram of body weight. So in order to work out the approximate quantity needed for each feed, multiply the baby's weight by 150, and divide by the number of feeds per 24 hours (usually about 6, although it may be as many as 8). This should bring you somewhere between 60 and 120 ml per feed. Babies may take different amounts at each feed, however, so it's best to put a little more in the bottle until you become accustomed to his habits — you can easily throw out the rest.

If you started off breastfeeding, but want to change from breastmilk to formula (weaning), have a chat first with your child health nurse or lactation advisor about weaning methods, types of formula and bottle-feeding procedure. Don't wean your baby without help.

For advice on equipment, see Baby shopping tips, pages 18–19.

Basic rules for bottlefeeding

- Feed baby on demand, rather than by the clock.
- Glass bottles are easier to clean but plastic ones are lighter, and safer if dropped.

- Follow instructions for measuring and mixing formula, as it can cause problems for baby if too weak or too strong.
- Use boiled water for 12 months. (Some experts advocate boiling it for 5 minutes, others say boiled water straight from the kettle is fine.)
- Cool water before adding to formula, otherwise the heat can destroy the vitamins.
- Sterilise all equipment for the first 12 months is the advice from the Department of Health (although some books tell you 6 months only). Teats, like dummies, should be kept in a sterile container in the refrigerator.
- You can make up a day's supply of bottles (say 6) and keep them in the refrigerator. Shake well before giving to baby. Or keep the boiled water in a jug and make up as you go.
- Don't keep mixed formula or boiled water in the fridge for more than 24 hours.
- The quantity to prepare is based on baby's weight so keep up regular weighing sessions.
- Remember that baby's appetite can vary from feed to feed, so you may need to prepare a little more, just in case.
- Put the bottle in hot water to warm it.
- Best not to use the microwave for warming. It's said to destroy vitamins, and heats the milk unevenly, continuing to heat when the bottle is removed, with the risk of burning baby's mouth.
- If you do microwave on occasions, at least make sure you remove the teat and cap (believe it or not, bottles have been known to explode, and microwaved teats to melt down into baby's throat!). And shake the bottle well to ensure even heat.
- Test milk temperature on the inside of your wrist.
- Feeding will usually take 20–30 minutes. If you hold the bottle upside down, and the milk flows, rather than drips out, then it's coming out too fast.
- Never leave baby to feed himself with the bottle propped up as he may choke.
- Throw out any milk that's left in the bottle after the feed. Don't leave it any longer than 15 minutes.

- Rinse empty bottles straight away, before washing. Turn teats inside out to clean, and squeeze water through the hole. You can buy special brushes for teats.
- When travelling, don't keep warm formula in insulated packs for more than 30 minutes or so, as this becomes a breeding ground for bacteria — insulate cold bottles instead. Better still, fill bottles with boiled water (which can be warm), and mix in the formula when it's time to feed. You can buy formula dispensers with three sections for pre-measured feeds, or pre-measured sachets of formula.
- Don't keep opened tins of formula more than a month.
- Don't feed cow's milk to baby until 12 months (they used to say 9 months). It's too high in protein and salt, and can result in iron deficiency and dehydration, amongst other things. However, boiled cow's milk can be used for mixing cereal or cooking after 6 months.

Sterilisation of feeding equipment

In the old days they used to boil bottles to sterilise them. Next, they would 'Milton' them. Then, in the nineties, they brought out steam sterilisers.

Milton is a chemical sterilising solution which you make up every morning in a special plastic container. If you're bottlefeeding you'll need a large container; if you're breastfeeding you can buy a smaller container (handy for dummies, the odd bottle and breast pump). After cleaning your equipment, submerge it in the solution for an hour. You may be tempted to rinse the last drops of the clinical-smelling solution from the bottle before filling it with milk or formula, but this defeats the purpose, as the bottle will no longer be sterile (anyway, the solution is said to be harmless and the baby apparently doesn't taste it).

For most bottlefeeding mothers, however, the steam steriliser is a dream, even if it does cost more. You simply put the clean equipment into the unit, add water, switch it on and it switches off automatically when finished. Job done, without the use of chemicals. You can also buy a microwave steam unit, which looks like a large microwave oven dish. It takes only 9 minutes. Check first with a health professional as to which model is currently recommended.

If you're breastfeeding, and don't have a huge amount of items to sterilise each day, you may prefer to boil for 10 minutes — although I know a few women who got sick of burning their fingers! — or use Milton.

Remember, once a boiled or sterilised dummy goes into the baby's mouth, then it's no longer sterile. If you use dummies, the best rule is to change them after each feed, or if the dummy drops onto the floor. You can store sterilised dummies in a plastic container in the refrigerator for 24 hours. It's best to have at least two so you can rotate.

Bathing tips

- You don't have to use expensive baby bath lotions or even mild soap — just some moisturising sorbolene cream in warm water is fine (try massaging baby with sorbolene before the bath). Baby powder isn't necessary.

- If you don't feel confident about testing the water (with your elbow or the inside of your wrist is best), you can buy floating temperature gauges.

- Deep water baths are much more relaxing, great for soothing unsettled babies. Baby should have only his head above the water, with your arm supporting his neck and underarm. If he's only half-immersed, he may get cold.

- If you choose to buy a plastic baby bath, find one deep enough for baby to float. (The contoured baths, which often come as part of a change-table set, are too shallow for this — and the contours are redundant, as you still need to support baby yourself.) More importantly, get one with a plug! That way you can rest it on the bench, and empty it by sliding it to the sink, rather than having to lift.

- If your poor back can't stand the strain of lifting a plastic tub filled with water onto a bench or change table, or bending over a bathtub while trying to balance a slippery baby, try bathing your newborn in the bathroom basin or kitchen sink — but make sure it's clean! Otherwise, use your laundry sink (nice and deep), with the washing-machine top serving as a change table. It beats

carrying buckets of water to the baby bath and, afterwards, all you have to do is pull out the plug. No lifting required.
- Don't worry — your plastic baby bath will come in handy later as an ice bucket, or a sink to wash dishes in when camping!
- Remember to turn on the answering machine or take the phone off the hook!

Nappy time

Despite all the lotions and potions available, the theory these days is 'the less, the better'. Cottonwool balls and warm water are really all you need at nappy changing time. Or you may choose olive oil, or sorbolene and glycerine cream (in a handy dispenser which saves you fetching warm water, and cleans and moisturises in one go).

You may like to apply a thin layer of Vaseline or zinc and castor oil cream to guard against nappy rash.

Change baby at each feed, and when necessary.

Nappy liners can be useful with cloth nappies. There are two types, disposable and cloth, so experiment to see which you prefer. Some are designed for sensitive skins, and draw more moisture away from the baby (helping prevent nappy rash); others aim at keeping the nappy cleaner and helping you dispose of the contents.

If no-one has thought to treat you to a month's nappy wash service, now's the time to ring and do it yourself (unless you prefer to use disposables for the first few weeks). You have better things to do right now than cope with soaking, washing and drying dozens of nappies.

Nappy rash tips

Nappy rash is caused by ammonia, from stale urine, and thrives on a combination of moisture and heat, so the basic rule is to keep baby dry.
- Change baby frequently.
- Rinse baby's bottom when changing, and dry well.
- Don't use nappy wipes, which may irritate the skin.

- Give baby time on the floor without his nappy whenever there is an opportunity.
- Curash powder, sprinkled on at each nappy change, is said to be effective in clearing up the rash.
- Use zinc and castor oil cream as a barrier (but make sure baby's skin is dry before you apply it). Plain zinc cream will stay on longer.
- One-way cloth nappy liners will help keep the urine away from his skin.
- Use super-absorbent pilchers, preferably the fluffy cotton ones. Never use plastic pants.
- Wash cloth nappies in natural soap flakes. Avoid bleach and conditioners.

Telephone help lines

One of the most important things to remember is that you can always call for help when it gets too much. Many women wait too long before they make that vital phone call, if they make it at all. But there's no reason to feel guilty or inadequate if you find you can't cope: all you need is the right advice to suit your baby. It's amazing how a little enlightenment from a seasoned carer can transform your life.

There are family care organisations in each capital city. They are staffed by trained nurses, and offer all kinds of support to mothers and babies, including day stays, week stays, home visits and 24-hour telephone counselling lines. The Nursing Mothers' Association of Australia also provides a 24-hour help line, as well as sessions for pregnant women and new mothers. So if you're at the end of your tether at 3 a.m., ring one of the 24-hour help lines available in your state. There are times when a good chat may be all you need, for comfort and reassurance.

Be aware, though, that some of these lines may be congested when you ring, especially during the night when there may only be one counsellor on telephone duty. You could get the engaged signal for hours, or be logged on by an answering service, and have to wait until you're called back. Have the numbers of several hotlines on hand, to avoid frustration. (See Help lines, pages 238–41.)

A father's view

The first week at home

Bringing a baby back home is a great occasion, the type of thing fathers are pretty good at (you know, over the threshold and all that). It's also a time when you become 'real parents' and leave all those helpful (but rather routine driven) nurses and carers behind. You will feel the thrill of the new as you (oh-so-carefully) drive away.

You are embarking on a great adventure

Like all adventures, there are many dangers and challenges in store, as you carry your newborn into your world (or rather what your world used to look like). Within a day or so, those bossy nurses are going to look like arch angels. Now there's nobody there to whisk this screaming red thing away and replace it moments later with a sleeping angel. That means this charming little bundle is not only going to deprive you and your partner of many hours sleep, but will put some significant strains on your relationship.

Extra-large doses of compassion and understanding are now required from all fathers. You may be used to working a 12-hour day, or running a large company, but this is a totally new, illogical, demanding and much more strong-willed opponent.

Your baby may cry every time you pick him up

It's not you! Even your own child may need time to get used to you in this strange new world. Even after a few days he might get startled and turn red and show off his tonsils. Don't pass him back like some hot potato; be brave and solve the problem yourself. Observe what your partner or carers do to soothe the child. You'll find it will do the trick for you as well. You are now a valuable member of the team.

Take a week off work
This is a great time to experience the joys of having a family. You'll feel a great deal of inner satisfaction and pride and find yourself exchanging knowing glances with your partner as it suddenly sinks in what a wonderful thing has happened. Just being together is the best. So don't miss it.

Don't be afraid to get involved
Far from being a male exclusion zone (full of strange tools like bottles, bibs, baubles and potions), caring for baby can be a proving ground — with a bit of practice, you will soon be able to whisk the baby away and masterfully change, soothe and re-present the joyous bundle to its mother. Being involved will make you feel that you are at last a partner, not just the awkward messenger. You both have a lot to learn, and the best way to do it is to get involved right from day one. This is the beginning of something special.

Helping with the night feeds
No matter how tempting it is to feign unconsciousness and will yourself back to sleep at the 2 a.m. feed, there is a lot to be said for offering support to your partner, even if she's breastfeeding. Company at that lonely hour is pretty special. It also helps you appreciate how the feeds can disrupt your sleep. Mind you, there's nothing better than gazing down on your baby during a feed — it is a special moment that fathers should not miss out on. The excuse that you have to get up soon and go to work cuts little ice with a mother who 'works' a 20-hour day.

Split the tasks
If you are one of the many who find it exhausting adapting to this 24-hour regime, try splitting the tasks rather than doubling-up on everything. It may mean you sleep through the night and early morning feeds, but can then help put the house back in order and let your partner catch up on much needed sleep through the day. This may increase the amount of control, rest and sanity in your household.

Checking on the baby

I hate to say this, but chances are for the first week or so you will wake bolt upright in the middle of the night because you heard your baby sneeze, or because you didn't hear him sneeze. You will find yourself creeping over to the cradle (heart pounding) just to check that everything is all right. Mind you, this will probably be just after you have lectured your partner about being paranoid. You will find yourself watching a sleeping baby just as intensely as your favourite program on television. (You remember the television, that large black thing in the corner that some people you know look at.)

Where do fathers turn for advice?

Well, we are meant to be resourceful. You will find few publications or organisations that cater to the 'other half'. (Yes, we can feel victimised here.) Your best ports of call are probably other fathers and bits of information accidentally included in baby books. If it all gets too much, go and wash the car or mend something you broke when it all got too much.

You may find yourself arguing vehemently over who had the bread knife, tea-towel, sleep disorder, last. I'm afraid it's just you both letting off steam while trying to cope with a huge change in lifestyle. It doesn't get much easier over the next few weeks but the quality of the arguments will certainly improve. The best solution is to laugh at it all right from the start and get back to the more important tasks.

Love

It's quite amazing. When you are in love with someone you assume that you are drawing upon limited reserves of love — it's full-time and full-on. But when this amazing creature joins your circle it untaps so much more — it seems like you have discovered an eternal spring. Where does it all come from? If you had a hundred children you would still have love in reserve. One of life's delightful mysteries.

2 WEEKS OLD

MILESTONES

- Can focus up to a distance of 20–30 cm.
- Uses hand to help hold dummy (involuntary reflex).

WHAT THEY NEVER TELL YOU THIS WEEK

- Most new babies cry more than you expected and sleep less.

- Motherhood doesn't come naturally to all of us — there are skills that must be learned.

- Be flexible. Don't be too worried or guilty if you haven't fed exactly on time or got him to sleep on time. The baby has to fit into your routine too.

- You don't have to tiptoe around the house while baby's asleep. It's best for him to adapt to normal noise levels.

- If you have problems coping, you can ask to be referred to a family care centre.

- Combining breastmilk and formula may be a last resort for some breastfeeding mothers.

- You may feel stressed and edgy, or sometimes burst into tears.

- You may squabble with your partner or fly off the handle.

THINGS TO DO THIS WEEK

- Visit your local child health centre.
- Start baby's individual book of milestones.

CHAPTER THREE
─────────
2 weeks old

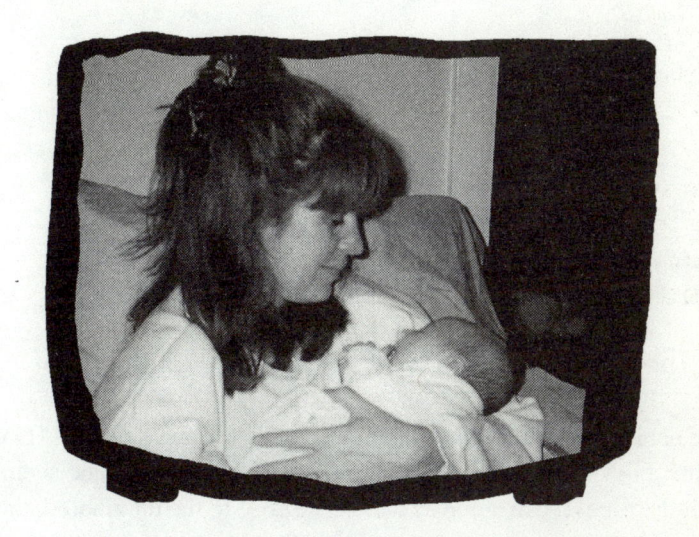

DAY 14

> *I had foolishly told my parents that Tristan and I wanted to be alone with the baby for a couple of days after returning home, thinking that we would really appreciate the privacy and the chance to establish our new family routine. They had come to Sydney from Melbourne while I was in hospital, and were staying with friends, so as not to intrude.*
>
> *Obediently, they didn't pay us a visit until today — and better saviours we couldn't have asked for. They ploughed into the pile of housework, washing and cooking, while we looked after the baby — all our Christmases had come at once! The unfortunate part is that Mum and Dad have already been in Sydney much longer than*

expected, due to Rupert's late arrival, and so have to return home in a few days' time. But not before making order out of chaos, stocking up our freezer with home-made soups and stews and saving our sanity — for a while longer at least.

> ## Your baby this week
>
> If your baby has seemed like a little crying/feeding/sleeping machine, albeit a lovable one, from now on things will change rapidly. Every week you'll notice new expressions, and new things your baby can do. Keep your own diary or baby book — and start it now, before you forget special moments. It's lovely to be able to look back on this precious time, and relive your excitement with your partner and child, when he is old enough to appreciate it.

They never said he was going to cry all the time!

Some babies are little dolls who lie peacefully for hours on end. (Don't you just envy their mothers?) But most babies cry and some seem to cry all the time. It can come as a huge surprise to the uninitiated, those who anticipated some pools of tranquillity throughout the day, the baby gurgling happily while they go about their chores. But don't worry, this may still happen later.

Babies may cry because they're hungry, wet, cold, need burping or have some other form of discomfort. They may cry because they're overtired. Or they may cry for seemingly no reason at all, and stubbornly refuse to be soothed, which is the most baffling, frustrating and upsetting experience for a new parent, especially if it continues for hours. (See Colic, page 74.) It makes parents, so much in control in our previous lives, feel guilty and ineffectual to see all our efforts fail, and have to helplessly stand by and watch our baby in distress. Not to mention what it does to our nerves!

The only good news is that most crying is normal, and sounds worse than it is. A good cry is often what a baby needs to let out the emotions of the day and get to sleep.

The art of settling

Ideally, you should establish a settling routine that both you and your partner follow each time baby is due to go to sleep. This way, baby knows that when you do this, it means he can relax ready to go to sleep. Don't try lots of different things — you may just confuse baby. That said, your old tried and tested routines don't always do the trick, so you have to have other strategies at the ready. Find out which of the settling techniques and aids work best for you, and stick to these as much as possible.

If baby wakes up crying, and you feel he hasn't had enough sleep, don't pick him up immediately — try letting him cry for a few minutes, in case he resettles. Tired babies who wake during their sleeping cycle often fall back to sleep if they're left alone.

Settling aids

- cuddling
- rocking chair
- baby pouch
- baby hammock
- baby swing
- pram ride
- car ride
- deep warm bath
- massage
- singing
- music
- sound of vacuum cleaner
- sound of washing machine
- sucking (dummy)
- pre-warm mattress (hot-water bottle)
- swaddling firmly

Settling to sleep

- Pat baby firmly and rhythmically on back or bottom, at 2-second intervals.
- Rhythmically rock or jiggle the bassinet.
- Allow baby to cry for a few minutes before coming back to pat, re-wrap or pop in dummy.

(See Controlled settling, pages 117–18.)

Don't be too precious about sleep time

Because it can be such a chore getting baby to sleep, and such a welcome relief for you when it happens, it's easy to start thinking of sleep time as a sacred period which must be respected at all costs. You may tend to creep around, take the phone off the hook, ask people not to ring the doorbell, or refrain from doing the vacuuming (who's got time to vacuum anyway!). It's probably better to make as much noise as you wish, so that baby becomes used to normal noise levels. This may mean he'll learn to sleep through anything! In fact, droning noises like the washing machine, vacuum cleaner or the radio usually act as great soothers.

Many mothers feel they have to wait until baby wakes up before taking him out, for fear of disturbing him. However, babies are very adaptable, and yours may well sleep on regardless. I always preferred to take advantage of that precious sleep time by staying home to do some of the many chores on my list. More sensible mothers would take a nap instead.

Who said it was easy?

By now you've realised that all the gruelling work associated with a new baby has been a well-kept secret. Why do other mothers make it look or sound so easy? Were they too embarrassed to reveal that they, too, had trouble coping at first?

The truth is that you are now dictated to by an unrelenting little tyrant. You can't arrange anything for a specific time and be sure of keeping the appointment, even within the same day. If the baby decides he's hungry just as you're about to walk out the door, you have no choice but to feed him. If you're breastfeeding, no-one else can do the job for you, so bank on being an hour or two late! Dirtying nappies or posseting on a fresh outfit are also foolproof ways of holding you up.

Gone are the days when meals were cooked and eaten at a set time. You may find you're skipping meals, or eating dinner at 11 p.m. You'll learn to like cold food, and become adept at eating with one hand. (Always have something in the freezer which you can heat up in the microwave.)

First-time mothers have a tendency to want to do everything perfectly and worry that they may be jeopardising the baby's well-being by not doing something according to the book. Just remember to temper all this dedication with some flexibility. If he's still sleeping when he should be feeding, or if you're in transit when you should be putting him down, then it's not the end of the world — babies have a remarkable tendency to survive. There's a limit to how much upheaval *you* can take (and still remain sane) but months later you'll look back on this time and wish you'd been easier on yourself.

When a friend of mine was feeling guilty that she was not being a good enough mum, her doctor told her that every time she felt this way she should ask herself three questions: 'Is my baby loved?' 'Is my baby happy?' 'Is my baby thriving?'. And, of course, the answer to all three was 'yes'.

DAY 17

Today he was awake and whingeing for a record 13 hours — from 9 a.m. to 10 p.m. I rang the Nursing Mothers' Association, and called Tristan several times, tired and tearful. Concerned, he came home early from work to find a tracksuit-clad wreck of a wife.

The mood was catching, and soon we were both weary and grumpy. Tristan resorted to putting Rupert over his shoulder and taking measured, rhythmical steps up and down the corridor. Someone had told us how ancient tribes successfully used the natural walking rhythm to calm even the most upset baby. But after 2 hours Rupert was still bellowing as Tristan methodically retraced his tracks, every inch of wallpaper and speck of dust an all-too-familiar sight. Then, for no apparent reason, Rupert fell asleep. ('Babies don't fall asleep — they plummet', a child health nurse once observed to me.) We lost no time following suit!

Relaxation tip

When it all gets a bit much, or you see red, stop everything for just one minute. If you're holding baby, put him down in a safe place, and walk into another room (or outside, into the fresh air). Close your eyes, take a deep breath, feel your limbs flop, and just focus on your breathing. This will instantly relieve your stress and put things back into perspective. If baby is asleep, and you have 5 or 10 minutes to spare, do the exercise lying on your back on the floor. This is a great refresher.

Get out and about

It's easy in the first few weeks to get bogged down in trying to do everything the 'right' way, and keep the house under control at the same time. But get out at least a couple of times during the week, even if it's just a walk around the block with baby in the pram or sling. At least this helps keep your weight under control. If you can afford it, join a gym with a child-minding service. Organise to have some regular contact with other adults to avoid losing your perspective — you may even get to have a laugh!

For some new mothers, the thought of having to tackle the intricacies of the baby capsule or pack a baby bag with everything that may be needed for half an hour away from home can seem insurmountable. Even bringing out the pram may be a daunting prospect if you live in an upstairs unit, or have difficult access to the street. Then, of course, there's getting yourself dressed and presentable to the outside world. (Vanity becomes a thing of the past!) Yet once you've made the effort, just escaping from the clutter and chaos that is probably your home at the moment gives you a new outlook, and is guaranteed to make you feel better.

Even a trip to the supermarket can be therapeutic, putting you back into contact with 'normal' life. (Find a supermarket that has baby capsules attached to some of the trolleys.) But beware — a newborn baby is sure to be the star attraction wherever you go, with strangers coming up to smile and coo.

For the ultimate treat, try a baby-sitter. Although it may be far too early for you to consider entrusting your new charge to a stranger, you could ask a friend or relative to hold the fort while you slip out for half an hour or so. An uninterrupted coffee, or stroll around the shops, could just make your day!

Child health centre

If you're living in an area serviced by a child health centre, now is a good time to pay them a visit to discuss how you and the baby are doing. The trip outside will do you the world of good, not to mention the advice and reassurance you'll receive from a trained carer.

The centres normally cater for babies and children from birth to 5 years. As well as being able to visit regularly for one to one consultations, you'll find a wealth of information available in the form of pamphlets, booklets, notice boards, and other mums. And nobody cares if your baby screams the whole time! By the way, fathers are not banned, so if your partner is home for a week or two, suggest he come along and share in the learning experience.

Visits are usually recommended at about 2 weeks (earlier if you have problems), 8 weeks, 4 months and 9 months, for growth and development checks as set out in your baby's personal health record. However, you can visit as often as you like for support and advice. The nurses will help you with feeding, crying, settling, and when to introduce solids — all the issues involved in parenting (right through to when your child goes to school).

At this first visit, the nurse will give baby a thorough physical examination, looking at his skin, eyes, hair, hips, umbilical cord and general health, as well as his height and weight, and sleeping and feeding patterns. She will also chat to you about your own wellbeing and ability to cope, and inform you about local facilities, groups and activities which you may like to take advantage of.

It's important to be *honest* with your nurse. Some women try to put on a brave front, so as not to look foolish or ignorant. Remember that no problem is too small to talk about — these carers have heard it all! If they feel you need more input and support than they can give, they will be able to recommend a specialist or family care organisation in your area. If you play down your problems, you could miss out on vital help.

Many first-time mothers like to visit each week for the first couple of months, as there always seems to be something you need to ask. At each visit you'll be able to weigh your baby, and keep a record of his progress. You'll probably get quite a thrill from monitoring the increase in weight from week to week. From now on, many babies gain about a kilogram a month, or 250 grams a week — but it could be anything between 150 grams and 450 grams a week.

While you're there, enquire about new mothers' groups. Most centres hold a series of weekly sessions which you may be able to enrol in when the baby's just a few weeks old, and receive invaluable guidance on how to cope with common problems and different stages of development. It's a great opportunity to meet mothers with babies the same age as your own, swap information, and possibly form long-lasting ties. It's so reassuring to be able to talk to mothers with the same priorities and problems.

Exercise

It's convenient to forget about exercise when you have important things like crying babies and washing to deal with. But make every effort to spend at least 5 minutes a day doing a few of those exercises they taught you in hospital, otherwise you run the risk of still having a saggy tummy months later. Make sure you're doing the exercises which are right for you, as the wrong ones can be damaging. And program yourself to do pelvic floor exercises at certain times, like after the toilet or in the shower.

Exercise videotapes focusing on the tummy are good, because they help you do the exercises correctly for maximum benefit, keep you disciplined, and you can do them at a time to suit you (a challenge in itself). Before you invest, you may like to rent or borrow one, to see if it is something you will persevere with.

Community resources

How are you coping? If you need to talk to someone, don't hesitate to ring your child health centre or one of the help lines listed at the back of this book (pages 238–41). If you find yourself becoming angry, and feel you're in danger of harming yourself or the baby, ring immediately. They will understand and be able to help — or refer you to someone who can. Don't let partners or well-meaning friends or relatives pressure you into believing it's all your fault or that you are being 'silly' not coping. Even the smartest, most organised superhuman can be brought to the brink by a newborn.

If you need some hands-on advice on putting the baby to sleep, dealing with constant crying or other problems, there are family care organisations based in each capital city. Your local child health centre or clinic serves as the first port of call, and they can refer you to more intensive services in your area. They may suggest you take your baby along (free of charge) for a morning or day stay. When you see a technique demonstrated with your own baby (and working like magic), it's so much more effective than just reading about it in a book.

If you're really at the end of your tether, you may be referred for a week stay at a family care centre, bringing along your baby (and partner as well, if he can make it). As well as receiving help for your particular problems, and learning about all aspects of baby care from highly trained nursing staff, you'll probably have meals cooked for you (a blessing), no housework, and the opportunity to catch up on some sleep. And it's surprising how uplifting it is to find other normal, capable people in exactly the same boat. Many women put off seeking help because they think things will improve, but often waiting just exacerbates the situation.

So if you need help, ask for it. You'll find your community has a lot to offer.

DAY 19

My father-in-law popped in this afternoon and joined Rupert and I in a visit to a private childcare centre which has opened its doors only a block away from our flat. It's a beautifully restored, sunny cottage with a neat back garden, run by Rhonda, a cheery, energetic woman with two young children of her own.

'Yes, we do take babies', she said, clucking at Rupert, cosy in his sleeping bag with hood. I was delighted as it can be hard to find centres which accept babies younger than 6 months. And this one also has extended hours (8 a.m. to 6 p.m.) to cater for working parents. I explained that I wanted to put him in for one day a week at first. She said she'd be pleased to welcome the youngest member of her 'family' and would enrol me immediately, as her lists were almost full.

What a find! Most people wait ages to get into a centre, especially one with good hours. And I had stumbled on to a great place right on my doorstep.

Now that I'm committed to day care (even if for only one day a week), I have to find some information on expressing milk. Because I plan to continue breastfeeding until at least 6 months, I'll need to learn how to express and store milk for the days Rupert is in day care.

Breastfeeding ease

Not everyone adapts easily to breastfeeding, so if you're still having problems, do talk to a professional about it before you give up. It's best to actually visit someone, whether it be an early childhood nurse, lactation consultant, or a member of the Nursing Mothers' Association, in order to get practical support. Or have a lactation consultant or mothercraft nurse visit you.

Breastfeeding can be hard on the back, so make sure you find a position where you're well supported. This may involve resting your feet on two telephone books, or placing two pillows on your knee to rest the baby on. Always place a pillow under your arm for support and try to keep your shoulders and neck relaxed.

Some women prefer to do night feeds lying on their side in bed. Others use a big boomerang pillow to lean back against. Whatever works best for you.

If you haven't enough milk

Women who aren't producing enough milk to satisfy their baby are often in a quandary as to whether to give up or persevere. After they've spoken to a few experts from different camps, they're liable to be even more confused. One desperate mother told me she had gone as far as to consult a paediatrician, lactation consultant, doctor, child health centre and a child and family nurse — and came away with a heap of contradictory advice.

A close friend of mine was also in a dilemma. Her paediatrician insisted she top up each breastfeed with formula, because the baby wasn't getting enough milk, while her lactation consultant strongly advised her not to offer formula, but instead to breastfeed more frequently to stimulate her own supply.

Both women became so stressed that they eventually stopped listening to others and decided to do what they thought was best. The controversial solution that finally worked for both was to alternate breastmilk and formula.

If you're wondering whether you should do this, do see a health professional first. Most will advise you not to introduce formula before 6 weeks if at all possible, in order to give your milk supply a chance. If you do have to offer complementary feeds, the general rules are to do it after the breastfeed, preferably just at times when your own supply is low, and to offer only a small amount of formula. So, go ahead and do what's practical for you and your lifestyle. The odd bottle of formula while breastfeeding doesn't seem to hurt; despite the grave warnings, it appears that most babies can go from formula back to breastmilk with no trouble. But try the baby with a bottle first (be it formula or breastmilk), before leaving him with a baby-sitter, just to make sure he'll take the teat.

Some experts get quite pedantic on the issues of alternating breast with teat, or breastmilk with formula, and can scare you into being too afraid to divert from the straight and narrow. Some say never to give your partner or baby-sitter formula to administer if you're away, only expressed milk. One reason is that formula may cause allergies in some babies. Others warn that introducing a bottle (even if it's filled with expressed milk) can lead to baby refusing the breast in favour of the freer flowing teat.

If you replace a breastfeed with formula, you may still have to express milk in place of the missed feed, for the health and comfort of your breasts. However, you won't have the pressure of having to express a certain amount by a certain time. Some mothers don't even worry about storing it — although I have to admit, I could never throw away good breastmilk. If you're expressing it anyway, put it in the freezer so baby can benefit.

When baby is a bit older, some breastfeeding mothers choose to substitute one or two feeds a day with formula on a regular basis, either because they have to go back to work, or simply to allow themselves a more flexible lifestyle. Others find this works well at the end of the day, when exhaustion has set in and milk is not as plentiful. This also gives other members of the family a valuable opportunity to establish the intimate rapport with the baby that comes with feeding.

As for how long to breastfeed, the general consensus seems to be that you should try to continue for at least the first 3 to 6 months, preferably aiming at 9 to 12 months, to give your baby the very best protection against infections and allergies.

DAY 20

Time to take Rupert to one of his father's clan gatherings. Today's family lunch was the first glimpse of the baby for Rupert's new aunts, uncles and cousins, so he was excitedly handed around while we bathed in the reflected admiration.

Rupert had soon had enough of the 'pass the parcel' game and loudly voiced his discontent. It's amazing how protective you get when you're a mum. I worried that he was becoming too tired and upset, and finally retrieved him for some peace and quiet. I had read somewhere that stress and fatigue could be contributing factors to cot death, so I was determined not to subject him to any undue strain. I was very possibly overreacting. But as much as I try not to think about it, the threat of cot death often lurks in my mind. I'll rest much more easily after the first 6 months.

The rest of the day passed enjoyably, the highlight being a big family roast. Rupert settled, and I found it was wonderful to have all those willing helpers: Tristan and I could actually enjoy warm food for a change, and eat with both hands!

Pass the parcel

It's about now that all your friends and relatives will be trooping through the house to inspect the new bundle (if they didn't last week). Or you'll be out and about showing off your pride and joy. You might get more than you bargained for.

Being flexible is one thing, but if you feel obliged to bring out the baby, even if he's sleeping, you run the risk of seriously disrupting your routine, and tiring both yourself and him. Sometimes you just have to be firm — they can look but not touch. If he's awake everyone's going to want to hold him — the poor baby may get passed around for 5-minute stints, often upset and bewildered by all the strange faces, not to mention the awkward positions in which he may be held. In all the excitement, you may not notice he's becoming overtired. Then you'll pay later, with an overstimulated and unsettled baby.

It's up to you where to draw the line. If it's upsetting you and the baby, call a halt to inspection time, and take charge of your charge.

Look after yourself

- Now that you've been going without sleep for a couple of weeks, you'll really be feeling tired, physically and emotionally. So promise yourself this week to take a nap as soon as you get the baby down — whatever the chores awaiting you. Chores will wait but a nap opportunity will fast disappear. And you need to re-charge your batteries during the day to deal with the unsettled periods that often occur in the late afternoon (commonly called the 'witching hours' in baby circles).

- Remember to eat. Skipping meals is no good when you need all the energy you can muster. Make time to prepare food, even if it means leaving baby to cry for a bit.

- If you need any more justification to give yourself a break, bear in mind that looking after yourself will help you care better for your baby. You'll have more stamina, and more patience, to meet his demands. A hungry, tired mum is often an irritable one, with a short fuse.

- If you've been cooped up in the house trying to cope for the last week, now's the time to get out into the sunshine, and endeavour to bring some normality back into your life.

A father's view

Well done! You have survived the first two weeks. You are now almost an expert in bottles, bathing, burping and beaming (that's what you do whenever you think about this amazing little bundle before you).

Nappies: the awful truth
Be warned — men seem to get to change all the really 'bad' nappies. Common decency prevents me going into any great detail. Women may never forget the agony of childbirth but men never forget that first nappy!

Cooking
By now you have probably used up all the pre-prepared meals, and if you do get to eat it is often on the spur of the moment (like cornflakes at midnight). The most helpful thing you can do is take over the kitchen one night (at least) and cook a real meal. You may be a little rusty, but it will taste like a million dollars and seem like the ultimate luxury for your partner (especially if you do the washing up too).

Doing it tough?
After another week of trying to cope with little sleep, and wondering how someone so small can take over your whole life, I asked my father how he had coped. When he told me that he had brought up six kids (three in nappies at the same time) in a small flat in London with the bath a 24-hour nappy washer and the ropes crisscrossing the kitchen as a clothes line, I was stunned into silence. I vowed never to complain again.

3 WEEKS OLD

Milestones
- May try to lift head while on tummy.
- Developing awareness.

WHAT THEY NEVER TELL YOU THIS WEEK

- You may still feel worn out and unable to cope.
- You may still be bleeding (that's quite normal).
- It may seem impossible to find time to do all your chores, let alone time for yourself.
- You may not yet feel up to resuming sex (but why doesn't someone tell your partner this?).

- Baby may develop common ailments such as milk rash or cradle cap.
- Overstimulating the baby during night feeds can rob you of precious sleep.
- Bleeding may stop, only to resume again in a week or so. This may be mistaken for a first period.
- Your period may resume any time within the next 9 months (often it's not until you finish breastfeeding).

THINGS TO DO THIS WEEK

- Schedule some time for yourself.
- Keep a diary of baby's routine.
- Check out your local childcare centres.

CHAPTER FOUR

3 weeks old

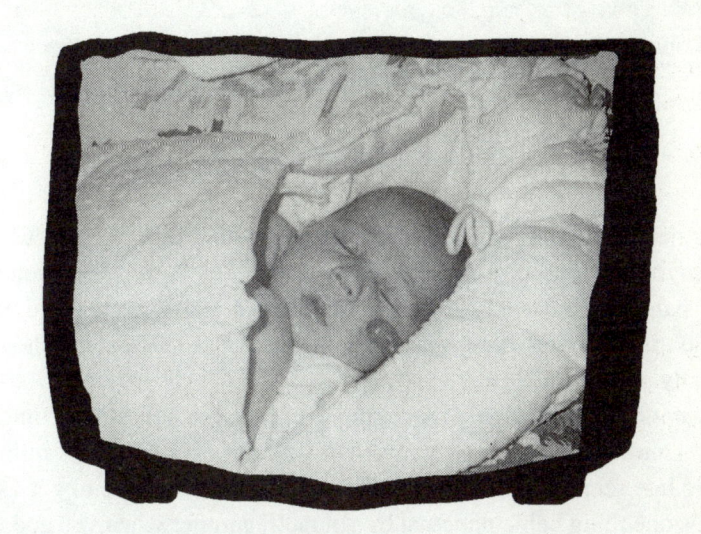

DAY 21

Rupert has a colourful clockwork clown mobile which hangs over the change table. When you wind it up the clowns rotate, playing the ubiquitous (but catchy) 'La La Lu' lullaby. Today he really noticed the clowns for the first time! He looked up and stared at them as they went round and round, flashing their wide red smiles. We had chosen this model (rather than a furry animal mobile which Tristan had set his heart on) mainly because of the smiles: someone had told me that the mouth and eyes, in real or symbolic form, are the first shapes a baby notices.

I'm glad I thought ahead when I was baby shopping during pregnancy and bought some clothes for 3 and 6 months. Rupert's growing so rapidly that he's already out of many of his smaller clothes — at only 3 weeks of age! He's obviously going to be tall, like his father.

WHAT THEY NEVER TELL YOU

Your baby this week

Watch for signs of your baby's developing awareness of the world around him. He may notice things he wasn't noticing yesterday. Make sure he has lots of moving things to attract his attention, like a string of dangling rattles on a frame. From now until 3 months, he will probably average 14–18 hours sleep a day.

The issue of time

They never tell you how little time (if any) you will have to yourself when you have a baby. No-one but a new parent could ever believe how babies manage to devour all your time and energy. Who else would believe you have mastered the art of a 30-second shower (usually at 3 p.m.)?

By now you're probably managing to escape the house from time to time. Don't be too hard on yourself if you're never running on time. Being late seems to be a fact of life all new mothers have to get used to. It's one thing being punctual by yourself, another when you add the random element of a baby who may decide to posset on your newly dry-cleaned suit as you walk out the door. Those who can maintain a sense of humour are most fortunate.

Schedule time for yourself

- Now is the time for a little reward, if you haven't treated yourself already.
- Book a masseur to come to your house (some specialise in prenatal and postnatal massage), while your partner minds baby in another room.
- Ask your partner to baby-sit while you go out for an hour.
- Take baby with you to the beautician and have a pedicure.
- Ask a friend to entertain baby, so you can catch up with things around the house.

Waking time activities

- Hang black-and-white mobiles over playmat or pram.
- Sit baby chair or bouncer on floor in front of a vertical mirror.
- Place an activity stand nearby and shake dangling toys.
- Go for a walk with baby in pouch.
- Talk to baby.
- Play him nursery rhymes or lullabies.

Baby pouches or slings

If you haven't yet purchased or used one of these invaluable items, now is the time to experiment. They're a bit fiddly to put on, but once you get the hang of it you'll be fine. A pouch really frees you up but remember, it should not be used for more than 1 to 2 hours at the most.

You can wear it around the house and have two hands free for your chores, while a grizzly baby is lulled by your warmth and movement. Or you can take a stroll around the block without having to bother with the pram. It's a good way to manage stairs and escalators while shopping, and it's convenient at the supermarket (although some smart supermarkets now have trolleys with built-in baby capsules). Make the most of the baby sling now as in a few months he may be too heavy for you to carry around for long periods. It won't be long before you can graduate to a backpack.

Baby swings and hammocks

In the more expensive category are the baby swings and hammocks, both on stands and both wonderfully effective soothers. Bear in mind that they take up quite a bit of space.

You can buy either a mechanical or battery-operated swing. Secure baby in the seat, wind it up, and let baby swing happily backwards and forwards while you have a few minutes free.

The baby hammock is often used in hospitals. Some nurses refer to it as the 'sin bin', because that's what crying babes are put in, much to the babes' delight! Make sure the hammock has adequate ventilation (mesh is good). And always position baby on his back.

To save money, friends of mine made their own baby hammock, attaching it by rope to a strong ceiling hook in a warm corner of the kitchen. They just gave a little push every few minutes while preparing the meal.

Home alone

Some new mothers have live-in relatives or a partner who works from home. Some have a whole network of family and friends living nearby, all willing to drop in and lend a hand. But many of us have to go it alone, during the day at least. This is hard going, and probably not the way babies were meant to be brought up.

This was only brought home to me when I compared notes with a friend who gave birth to her second child while living in rural Italy. She had no local family care centre or new mothers' group but she did have hoards of local village women and children who dropped in regularly, pleading to take the baby off her hands for an hour or two. Carol's theory, now that she's had two very different experiences of babyhood, is that babies are meant to be had in the bosom of extended families or social networks; it's when you're alone that exhaustion and despair can set in. Most households in her village comprise grandmothers, sisters, aunts and lots of other children, along with the parents themselves. Imagine the luxury of having four unsolicited 'breaks' of baby minding every day!

DAY 22

My goodness, it takes forever to get out of the house in the morning when you have a young baby — organising the bag with spare nappies, clothes, wipes, tissues and toiletries, organising the baby (changing nappies, and clothes that have been posseted on), trying to juggle your escape in between feeds and sleeps, then settling baby into capsule and loading up your other arm with the luggage. Phew! Only to find once you're at the car that you've left something behind — like a cap for his head when it's windy and cold or, even worse, the plastic bags to hold used nappies! Coupled with that you're tired, grumpy and slow-moving yourself, having been up for the 2 a.m. feed and awake since the 6 a.m. one. Is there ever any rest?

Developing a routine

The best time to settle baby at this stage is about $1\frac{1}{2}$ hours after the start of feeding, aiming at a 4-hour cycle of roughly $1\frac{1}{2}$ hours awake, and $2\frac{1}{2}$ hours asleep, so that baby sleeps a total of 14–18 hours.

After feeding, spend a little time with your baby, getting to know him and having a play. Then put him into his cradle to settle him down to sleep. Don't be afraid to let the baby cry or whinge alone for 3 to 5 minutes after you put him down: it may be heart-rending for you, but it's part of the normal settling process.

The routine you follow obviously depends to a large extent on you and your baby. For example, many babies, particularly those who are small or premature, will need feeding at 2- or 3-hour intervals. This is very demanding on you, especially during the night. With any luck, and a bit of sound advice, you should be able to extend those intervals within the next month.

Daily routine

Obviously babies don't function like clockwork, but it's handy to have a guide to aspire to, in some sort of attempt to organise your day. So your ideal feeding/sleeping routine, if your baby does feed approximately every 4 hours, could look something like this:

6 a.m.	Feed/change
7.30–10 a.m.	Baby sleeps (2$\frac{1}{2}$ hours)
10 a.m.	Feed/change/play
11.30 a.m.–2 p.m.	Baby sleeps (2$\frac{1}{2}$ hours)
2 p.m.	Feed/change/play
3.30–6 p.m.	Baby sleeps (2$\frac{1}{2}$ hours)
6 p.m.	Feed/change/play
7.30–10 p.m.	Baby sleeps (2$\frac{1}{2}$ hours)
10 p.m.	Feed/change
11 p.m.–2 a.m.	Baby sleeps (3 hours)
2 a.m.	Feed/change
3–6 a.m.	Baby sleeps (3 hours)

Night feeding tip

Sometimes it's tempting to have a little play in the middle of the night, during or after the feed, but this is no good for you or baby. Make sure you don't unintentionally stimulate him, or the feed will drag on too long. Avoid talking, smiling and eye contact — save all your communication for the daytime. Keep baby drowsy with hushed tones and dim lighting. (And resist any temptation to switch on the radio or television for your own entertainment!) After the feed, no playing — straight back to sleep.

Sex

You're now into your fourth week since the birth, and while some women will resume sex this week, others may be wondering just how much longer they can stall the advances of eager partners. You may still feel too tired, tender or simply disinterested. Don't feel it's your fault, or let yourself be persuaded that you're abnormal. Do what's comfortable for you. Some women prefer to wait until they visit their obstetrician for the 6 weeks checkup, and get the all clear to go ahead. It could well take up to 12 months before you feel totally at ease with sex again (as in the old days).

In any case, do communicate with your partner so there are no misunderstandings. He may be feeling left out and frustrated, and you can't afford to build up the tensions any more than they are already. Try to arrange some time to be alone. Get a baby-sitter and go out together. The baby will be fine, and you will both enjoy the break away from the pressures of being new parents.

And don't underestimate the importance of keeping up those pelvic floor exercises (those ghastly words again). Remember, your internal muscles have stretched considerably, and really need toning to be in good working condition.

---

13 reasons why you may not be feeling sexy

You're exhausted.

You're stressed.

You've got too much to do.

You're still bleeding.

You're still sore or tender.

You're nervous about penetration.

Your breasts are full and leaking.

Your breasts are now associated with feeding.

> Your body no longer seems your own.
>
> You're feeling flabby and overweight.
>
> You've been neglecting your appearance.
>
> You need sleep more than you need sex.
>
> You really do have a headache.
>
> (And even if you do try, the baby cries!)

Day stays

Don't feel uneasy about visiting a family care centre or day stay clinic if you have problems. It's free, it's one-to-one with a qualified, experienced carer, and it's amazing the difference just a few hours can make. You'll find people from all walks of life coming to cry on the nurse's shoulder, and swap stories and tips with other mothers. Babies are great levellers.

Many (but not all) family care services require a referral from a doctor or child health nurse. They will be able to advise you on what services are available in your particular area. Sometimes the waiting lists are long; the time you wait will depend on the urgency of your situation.

Having made the booking, you simply bring your baby to the centre with you on the assigned day, and go through your normal routine of feeding, changing, playing and settling, but under the supervision of your assigned carer. This way she can carefully observe you with your baby, and point out any areas that can be improved. Even the best baby book can't give you feedback or advice directed at your particular baby's needs — this is where professional help and one-to-one demonstration are invaluable. (More about family care centres on pages 135–6.)

DAY 23

My nearest day stay clinic is situated in a lovely old two-storey house in a tranquil leafy street, part of the network of Tresillian family care services. I was assigned to Kate, the child health nurse who would also look after me at any future visits. We sat down in the large, airy playroom, put Rupert on the floor on a rug, and talked about why I'd come — which was because I had been having trouble settling him, and was a nervous wreck as a result!

When it was time for a feed, Kate observed our technique, and answered my questions. Then came time for Rupert's sleep, and I witnessed nothing short of a miracle: Kate placed him on his side in one of the centre's white wicker bassinets. He was crying furiously, as he usually does when I put him down. I was resigned to the long, frustrating process of getting him to sleep, rocking the cradle from side to side for maybe half an hour. Instead, Kate started patting him surprisingly firmly and rhythmically on his bottom (through the padding of a nappy, of course). Immediately he stopped crying. While I watched in amazement, she jiggled (rather than rocked) the cot for another minute, eased off the patting, and he was fast asleep! The rhythmical nature of the patting was most important, she explained.

Kate gave me some other valuable tips: settle the baby about $1\frac{1}{2}$ hours after the start of feeding, aiming at a 4-hour cycle of roughly $1\frac{1}{2}$ hours waking, and $2\frac{1}{2}$ hours sleeping time; and don't be afraid to let the baby cry or whinge for 3 to 5 minutes after you put him down.

Controlled settling

This is advocated if the baby doesn't respond to your normal settling techniques. It simply means allowing the baby to cry on his own for a couple of minutes, before coming back for another try with your settling technique (but not picking him up). It's practised only after you feel you've met all your baby's other needs — that is, you've ruled out obvious causes of crying like hunger, wet nappy, overheating and cold — and the next thing on the agenda is sleep.

At first, most new mothers find it very difficult, if not impossible, to let baby cry unattended. You may feel callous, guilty or grief stricken. Some of us are hardy enough to walk away for a while; others (like me) huddle at the doorway, peeking through a crack, needing every ounce of willpower not to run to his side! Certainly it's easier to learn this technique when you have an experienced carer at hand, who can reassure you that you're doing the right thing, and demonstrate how it works. Crying, they say, is a natural part of the baby's settling process, and one which helps to tire him out ready for sleep.

It's certainly worth being brave and trying this technique. You'll probably be amazed at how quickly baby will respond when left to his own devices. The catch, of course, is that although sometimes baby will drift off to sleep like magic, other times he will keep on crying. You have to judge how long to allow it or how long you can bear it. Never leave baby to cry alone for more than 5 minutes, before coming in again to check, comfort, and attempt to re-settle.

Keep a diary

It's good to get into the habit of jotting down the times your baby sleeps and feeds. As well as giving you a better idea of baby's routine and progress, it provides a clear picture to show to any carer you may go to for advice. You'll find a diary useful to hand to a baby-sitter or nanny, so they can follow on where you left off.

Some common ailments

Milk rash
This is a red, blotchy, sometimes crusty rash, which often appears on baby's cheeks, and can look serious, although it's in fact harmless. Despite the nickname 'milk rash', it is not caused by milk, but by hormonal fluctuations which can result in a variety of oily conditions

— including rashes, pimples, pustules and cradle cap — conspiring to spoil baby's flawless complexion during the first few months. Usually no treatment is recommended.

Cradle cap
This is a scaly, greasy, yellow-brown rash which forms crusts on the scalp and eyebrows, caused by the baby's glands secreting too much oil. It can appear overnight, and cause great distress to new mothers who (wrongly) believe that it is caused by neglect. As it can look like baby's head is dirty, it can cause lots of embarrassment, especially to those who are ignorant of the condition. Surprisingly, many babies are affected within the first 6 months. It is certainly not your fault.

The way to deal with cradle cap is to remove the crusts each day until the condition clears up. Massage baby's scalp with olive oil or petroleum jelly, leave overnight, then wash briskly with soap and hot water, and towel dry. Brush scalp every day with a soft-bristled baby brush. If the crusts are on eyebrows or the skin behind the ears, massage with sorbolene and glycerine cream, and gently remove with a face washer when bathing. If it doesn't clear up in a few days, ask your child health centre or doctor to recommend a more effective preparation.

DAY 24

Just when you think everything's going well, it doesn't. One minute you're happy, the next minute tired and tearful. Rupert decided not to respond to my Tresillian settling method, household duties and dishes were piling up and workmen bustled in and out of the mess delivering a set of new windows to replace the leaking ones. Then Tristan arrived home and we started snapping again. It's so hard to avoid taking out the day's tensions on each other. When you have spent your life being very organised and efficient at home and at work, it's doubly frustrating that you can be thrown into such utter chaos by one tiny little being — whether awake or asleep — and not be able to do a thing about it!

> ### Crying tip
>
> When your baby cries, think of it as an effort to communicate, rather than a punishment for something you have or haven't done. Take a few moments to really be with him: listen to him, look into his eyes (if they're not too screwed up!). Then answer him by responding to what you interpret as his needs.

DAY 25

I felt sure I'd be able to get some work done today, with Tristan home to share the load, but it's amazing how Rupert seems to devour all our time. It doesn't seem possible (I pooh-pooed the notion when put to me by others in days long gone by), but somehow all we managed this afternoon was snatches of housework, meal preparation and bill payments in between bouts of feeding, pacifying and changing. There was no room for real relaxation, for either of us, and no time for me to work on the several projects vying for my attention. Tristan and I are both really feeling the effects of being overtired and housebound (housebound both because we have so much to do at home, and because we're too tired to go out — a vicious circle!). No matter how many resolutions we make, we still end up grumpy and snapping at each other. We both feel frustrated and deprived, and think one should be doing more to pamper the other.

Enrolling for childcare

By now, you're probably marvelling at how strong a hold this little creature has on your heartstrings. This is something no-one can imagine before the event — the power of this all-embracing instinct to love and nurture and protect; the reluctance to leave your precious charge in the hands of someone else. For some, going anywhere without their baby at this early stage is like cutting off a limb. A few hours at a day-care centre would seem like total abandonment.

Despite all these feelings, many mums now have to start thinking about local child-minding facilities.

It's certainly worthwhile checking out your local childcare options at this stage, if you haven't already. Some places don't take babies, and most have extremely long waiting lists (forward-thinking parents put their name on a list before birth!). Your local council will be able to supply you with the names of childcare facilities in your area, and information about their times and prices. Take baby for a stroll in the pram, and check out a different place each day.

If you plan to go back to work in 3 months, or even 12 months' time, you have to start planning now. In any case, your situation may change dramatically in 6 months' time. It doesn't hurt to at least put baby's name down on a list, to ensure you of a place in the future (although beware, most places will require a deposit to secure the reservation). It may seem inconceivable now to leave your precious cargo in the hands of a stranger, but once you've made contact and checked out the facilities, you may be greatly reassured.

Even if you're not planning to go back to work, there'll probably be times when you'll need to get out by yourself for an hour or more — to shop, have your hair done or do some exercise. If you haven't any relatives nearby, you could use occasional care for this. Or you might prefer to book baby into a childcare centre for one morning a week, to give yourself a regular break when you can get your own things done, or simply have a rest.

Childcare options

Day-care centres, preschools and kindergartens
These usually require regular bookings, even if it's only one day a week. Some take only preschoolers (3 to 5), some take babies and toddlers (babies to age 3), and some have a combination creche and preschool (babies to age 5). Long day-care centres, open from at least 8 a.m. to 6 p.m., cater for working parents. They're usually open for most of the year, although some close for school holidays. Council-run centres are cheaper than private ones, and may have longer waiting lists.

Occasional care centres
These cater for the parent who needs a break for a few hours or more, whether it's to go shopping, or attend an appointment. Usually you can't book a regular timeslot — you have to take pot luck on there being a vacancy when you ring, and there's a limit on the number of hours per month for any one child.

Family day-care or home-based care
This involves leaving baby with a selected carer, who looks after a small group of children in her own home, often including her own children. There is usually a limit of 4 or 5 children per group. Contact your local council or child health centre for details of home caregivers in your area.

Baby-sitting
If you want to take the evening off, it's not a crime to engage a baby-sitter at this early stage (indeed, for some it may be a sanity saver!). It's wonderful if you have willing grandparents, but if not, don't despair. Other people are capable of looking after your baby, despite what you may think. And they probably won't be offended if you ring every half hour to check he's still okay!

Of course, you can never be too careful when choosing a baby-sitter. Ask other mothers or your child health centre if they can recommend a reliable person or a reputable agency. Or, if you're desperate, choose a large established agency from the phone book. When your children are older, you can ask them how they liked the baby-sitter, or judge for yourself by their interaction, but with babies you have to go by a combination of reputation, gut feeling and good luck. (See also School and preschool, pages 229–30.)

A father's view

You have a gorgeous child, about to lose his 'newborn' tag. In a matter of weeks (maybe months) your baby will be sleeping through the night, parenthood will continue to become more manageable, and, of course, each new month will bring with it new joys.

Making eye contact with your baby
Even at this age your baby can focus on items up to a distance of about 20–30 centimetres. This means that the baby loves to see your face up close, as well as hear your voice. He may not approve of your dress sense, but at least he can't say anything.

Handling techniques
You may want to enjoy your new friendship in typical male fashion, by giving baby a taste of aerial adventure. After all he's bound to just love being tossed in the air. DON'T. You can easily damage and jolt tender young bodies and put things out of alignment. Always treat babies with the greatest care and respect. Give them rougher games when they are old enough to request such games themselves. Remember to always support the head and use that natural device — the crook of the arm.

Shopping techniques
Shopping for babies is expensive. How can one-third of a square metre of fabric with a few cute holes for arms and legs cost so much? This extra financial burden may mean you have to give up a few luxuries but the benefits are more than worth it.

Expect to become an expert at baby shopping. You will find yourself hanging around baby shops most weekends (I bet you never noticed them before) for the latest in baby wear and baby gadgets. High tech and good design (which we men can relate to) have finally hit the baby market but make sure the staff demonstrate that tricky new folding stroller first — it would be a shame to lose face.

Buy a bath thermometer. You'll get years of use from this one item and prove to your partner that you know all about baby's needs.

Keep the camera loaded

Like any good news journalist you will have to be always at the ready. Babies are not performing seals. That amazing physical feat, smile or sign of absolute genius may only appear once. So if you have a camera at hand you will have the best chance of capturing those magic moments. If you own a video camera, you'll like creating a priceless gift for your child. If you don't have one maybe a friend or relative could do some shooting for you.

Sex (and babies)

Just because your partner is about as interested in sex as you are in cleaning out the darkest recesses of the fridge, there is no need to abandon it altogether. You may have dropped a dozen obvious hints and even left your partner's finest knickers in very strange but highly visible places, but be patient. Sex will soon return to (almost) normal. Remember, neither of you is getting much sleep and that is hardly conducive to relaxed intimacy. Also, if the birth was a caesarean it's probably advisable to wait another week or two before gentle resumption. It may take up to 12 months to get totally back to normal.

What mothers always complain about fathers doing

It's not anything to do with the above. It's overstimulating the baby. You've come bouncing home from work full of energy and just dying to see your child. If he's asleep you will 'accidentally' wake him up. If he has just finished a feed, you will instantly want to play loud and raucous games, whereas the ideal situation (as your partner will probably hiss at you) is to let baby drift off to sleep, content and full. Otherwise you'll have a tired but wakeful baby that your poor partner has spent the last 6 hours desperately trying to get down.

Crying tips for helpful fathers

Your partner is in a state. Mother and child are tired, frustrated and in tears. This is the perfect time to try this magic trick. Take the baby and talk, sing or move around the house, and within seconds you may see a remarkable transformation or, at worst, you will know how they feel. The amazing art of distraction will, on many occasions, render that howling blob (and the baby) into a gurgling, happy bundle. Patting and walking also help. Remember to do your dues when the crying's on, to give your partner a desperately needed rest.

If you're back at work

After the excitement of the first week off after the birth, and slowly settling back into work on the second week, the third week away from the day-to-day dramas of home can begin a subtle separation between the parents. Your partner may find it hard to describe the blur of her daily events, just as your office talk may seem to her a trifle irrelevant. Make sure you put in the time to listen and share things with her and the baby. What worked for us during this time was a 5-minute face-to-face, no-distraction talk about ourselves and each other.

Losing friends

Having a child is a great way of discovering that some of your best friends aren't. For many of us fathers who have been engrossed in work-related socialising with other male colleagues, the arrival of the baby heralds the exit of some of your most dependable drinking/chatting partners. For some reason they are unable to find the same fascination with nappies, bottles and babies. Some may never come back but, like all things, there are many more to be made.

Pamper your partner

Bring home some flowers; buy a video camera; or have the latest roll(s) of happy baby snaps developed! She's going through a hard time — it's not only you who is feeling the strain. Listen, support and help. Do the chores unasked but don't be surprised if she doesn't want to drop everything and go out to dinner.

1 MONTH OLD (4–7 WEEKS)

MILESTONES

- Puts hand to mouth and sucks it.
- Lifts chin up while on tummy.
- Will hear a small bell rung 10 cm from his ear.
- Smiles at parents.
- May laugh aloud by the end of the month.
- May occasionally sleep through the night.

WHAT THEY NEVER TELL YOU THIS MONTH

- Your baby may have growth spurts, requiring more frequent feeds.
- Baby needs time on his tummy every day to help gross motor development.
- Sleeping through once at this stage doesn't necessarily mean it will happen the following night.
- Breasts can leak milk at inappropriate moments, so wear breast pads when you go out.
- You should not go swimming until bleeding has finished (which means the cervix is closed).

- Breastfeeding is *not* an infallible means of contraception.
- Storing and thawing breastmilk requires strict hygiene measures.
- Distraction may stop baby crying.
- If you feel continually anxious, depressed, angry or insecure, you may be suffering from postnatal depression.

THINGS TO DO THIS MONTH

- Enrol in a postnatal mothers' group if available.
- Catch up with members of your prenatal class.
- See your obstetrician for a 6-week checkup.
- Resume sex if you and the doctor feel you are ready.

- Consider forms of contraception.
- Start an exercise regimen.
- Remember your pelvic-floor exercises.
- Soak in a hot bubble bath with a magazine for half an hour, while your partner takes charge of the baby.

CHAPTER FIVE
===

1 month old (4–7 weeks)

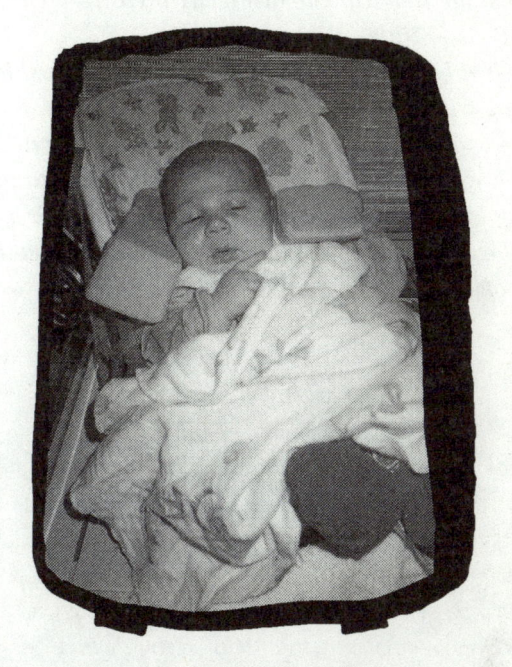

4 WEEKS

It was Father's Day and, rather symbolically, we made love for the first time since the birth. I still felt I wasn't quite ready, so it was a rather tense experience. But at least now we've broken the ice.

We decided that since this was such a special day, we would spend it together as a family, rather than visiting my father-in-law, as we usually do on Father's Day. We packed a picnic lunch, a chilled bottle of wine and Rupert's 'suitcase', put him in the pram, and strolled down to a nearby harbour-side park.

It was a lovely sunny day and many others had the same idea, stretching out lazily on rugs on the grassy hill overlooking the harbour. Rupert was wearing a white embroidered sun bonnet and his best blue velour jumpsuit. He looked really sweet. We perched near the edge of the embankment in the shade of a tree (carefully securing the pram with a rock as well as the brake) and laid out lunch while Rupert, lulled by the ride, drifted off to sleep. Later I leant against the tree trunk to discreetly breastfeed (first time in public, so I was a little self-conscious).

We walked back up the hill, legs aching from pushing the pram after so long without exercise. It had been a mellow, relaxing afternoon — so good for us to get out into the fresh air. How wonderful it would be to have a garden, to be able to lie with the baby on the lawn. Much as we love our apartment, it is just too small for the three of us. We really have to think about moving to a house soon.

Your baby this month

You can look forward to lots of exciting developments this month as your baby blossoms into a real little personality, with full-blown smiles, laughter, and the beginnings of vocalisation. Each week brings with it new wonders. He'll turn at the sound of your voice. His appearance will change as he puts on weight and fills out, and his eyes move closer to their final colour. Don't be surprised if you notice a sudden increase in his appetite as he goes through a growth spurt. He may start to skip a feed during the night.

Baby's neck is becoming much stronger, losing the newborn floppiness. He'll be able to lift his head up for longer while lying on his tummy and, if you pull him up to a sitting position, you'll see that head control is developing. But do continue to support his head until at least 6 weeks.

The 6-week point is a real milestone for most parents. The relentless drudgery of feed/change/cry/sleep eases, as baby becomes more settled, goes a bit longer between feeds, and a routine emerges. He may sleep an average of 14–16 hours, hopefully with the longest sleeps during the night. If you're breastfeeding, you'll notice that the milk supply is more stable, as your body now understands how much milk to produce. With baby sleeping a bit less during the day, and feeding more efficiently, there is more time for play.

Play

Maybe you haven't thought of playing with your baby — after all, you've been so busy coping with the basics! But now's the time to start giving up to half an hour's play in between sleeps, before or after feeding. Playing is important for baby's development.

Part of the play time could be spent with baby in a semi-upright position (portable chair or adjustable bouncer), with colourful baubles dangling from a wire stand to catch his attention. Why not play him some music, sing him some nursery rhymes, or read him a book (yes, even at this tender age!).

From 4 weeks onwards, at least 5 minutes of each play period should be spent lying face down. This vital part of baby's development is now commonly referred to as 'tummy time'.

Tummy time

'Tummy time', or lying tummy down, is said to be important for developing gross motor skills, and strengthening neck, back and arm muscles. However, the current emphasis on tummy time by many health professionals is a relatively new development, and you won't find it mentioned in your older baby books. This is because up until the early nineties, most babies were routinely put to sleep on their tummies, and so had plenty of opportunity in their cots to practise head lifting and raising body on arms.

Since SIDS research indicated the tummy-down sleeping position to be a risk factor, and changed their recommendations regarding sleeping posture, physiotherapists have noticed the adverse effects of babies being given insufficient time face down. For example, some babies 'bottom shuffle', instead of crawl, because they've spent most of their time in a sitting, or face-up position.

At 4 to 6 weeks, it's hard work for baby to keep his head up for long, and some babies will try to convince you they want out. But repetition is the way to get the strength he needs, so encourage or 'bribe' him to enjoy being face down on the floor for a short time between feeds, preferably with his nappy off.

Try 5 minutes on his tummy, followed by 5 minutes on his back. (Some babies tend to posset if you put them on their tummies straight after a feed, so you will have to judge for yourself when's the best time.) If baby's reluctant at first, you can ease him into the new position by giving him tummy time across your knees, or try lying on your back on the floor or bed with baby lying on top of you, tummy to tummy.

If he starts to grizzle, it probably means he's tired, so wrap him up and put him straight to bed before he becomes overtired.

Tummy-time treats

- Leave baby's nappy off so it's easier for him to lift his head (and also gives his bottom some fresh air).

- Put a rolled up nappy or bunny rug under his armpits to make him more comfortable.

- Lean a mirror up against the wall, so he can admire his reflection.

- Place an interesting toy, such as a chime ball, in his line of vision.

- Put baby face down on large blow-up beach ball, and gently roll forwards and sideways.

4 WEEKS

I had two full days of work scheduled for this week, so I needed to be well prepared. Over the last week I've painstakingly expressed enough breastmilk to supply Rupert with 2 to 3 feeds a day for his time at creche. What an effort! It was worst in the mornings — forcing myself to stay awake for an extra half-hour after the 6 a.m. feed, hands and wrists aching with the strain of pushing and pulling the pump — an awkward action at the best of times. And so little milk to show for it! Then making sure each portion is properly chilled and stored in sterile bags or bottles in the freezer. I had Rupert's frozen bottles already packed in a little 'lunch box', ready to transport with him.

This was the first time I had spent a whole day away from my baby. As I worked, my mind kept wandering: How is my little boy doing? I'll never forgive myself if anything happens to him while I'm away. How sweet he looked when I dropped him off.

As soon as morning tea break was announced, I rushed to a telephone and rang the creche. Yes, he was fine. But I wasn't — my breasts were beginning to feel uncomfortable and heavy, having missed the usual 10 a.m. feed. Fortunately I had brought my breast pump with me, and at lunch break locked myself in a room to express as much as I could in the limited time available. But I hadn't thought to bring an insulated container to keep the milk cool, so had to pour it all down the sink. What a waste!

Other than that, the day felt like a holiday: work was a breeze compared with the all-consuming responsibility of caring for a demanding infant. I really enjoyed being able to do something well, and getting praised for my efforts. And the freedom of being able to drink a cup of coffee or eat a sandwich, in surprising peace. Yet I couldn't wait to get back at 5.30 p.m. and take the baby into my arms again. My breasts were greatly relieved, too!

Sleeping and feeding patterns

Your baby's sleeping and feeding routine should become more manageable this month. For example, if you have been feeding every 2 to 3 hours, you may well make the transition to every 4 hours. If you are feeding as frequently as 2 a.m., 4 a.m. and 6 a.m., you may be able to drop one night feed by resettling baby without a feed. Aim to stretch baby to the time you want to wake up, whether it be 5 a.m. or 6 a.m.

If you're bottlefeeding, quantities are still measured roughly by 150 ml per kilogram of body weight, which means an average feed may range between 120–150 ml.

At this stage, baby may be sleeping 14–16 hours in 24. Give him as much sleep as possible. Waking periods during the day should ideally last 1½ to 2 hours (virtually the time it takes to feed, change and have a short play), then straight back to sleep.

(See Ideal routine, pages 113–14.)

5 WEEKS

Rupert smiled! At 5 weeks 2 days old. It wasn't the 'windy grimace' of a smile we've often seen, but a real smile, looking straight into Tristan's eyes (lucky him!). It was just after the 6 a.m. feed. Tristan was standing at the foot of the bed holding him up and talking to him. Suddenly Rupert's face lit up as he beamed back. What a wonderful moment. He looks like a real little boy now!

Just as I was thinking 'Ah, the 5-week mark — things have definitely improved', things deteriorated! First, Rupert wouldn't go down after his 2 p.m. feed. He stayed awake all afternoon, screaming until his face looked like a bellowing red beetroot. How inadequate it makes you feel! It's so hard not to see him as an 'ungrateful baby', treating you like this when you're doing everything in your power to make him happy and comfortable. Why doesn't he respond? Later in the evening I jiggled his cradle far more violently than Tresillian had ever taught. The poor little thing, it's a wonder he wasn't sea-sick! It's so hard to control yourself when you're driven to distraction. I realised what I was doing, and stopped, filled with remorse. But it had done the trick — he was asleep!

Bedtime routine

It's not too early to get into a special routine at bedtime. This will help baby differentiate between day and night sleeps, establishing familiar patterns which will help with settling in the future.

Perhaps you might bathe him every evening. Some parents find this helps to settle. Put baby to bed in his cradle or cot rather than letting him fall asleep in your arms or at the breast, so he comes to learn that bed means sleep. Perhaps you could play the same music each evening (there are some great relaxation and lullaby tapes available), or put the same toy in with him. If you spend the evening away from home, familiar toys or music will provide comfort and security.

Managing sleep

All our instincts say let the baby sleep. After all, he must need it, and we need the peace and quiet. But if baby sleeps for long periods during the day, waking up more frequently at night, the pattern has to be broken, for both your sakes. For example, if he goes for 6 hours between feeds during the day, it's recommended you wake him at the 4-hour mark, in order to encourage him to have the longest sleeps at night.

At this stage, he should be sleeping after each feed. If he misses a sleep, he may be too tired to feed effectively at the next feed, which may mean he's too hungry (and overtired) to settle and so the cycle continues. Even if you feel baby is happy staying awake, this could lead to troubles further down the line.

If you are having trouble solving problems to do with sleeping, feeding or settling, it's best to consult your child health centre or local family care service.

Tips for settling

- Try a warm bath if baby is unsettled.
- Pre-warm mattress with a hot-water bottle.
- Put baby to bed as soon as he shows signs of tiredness.
- Put baby down in his cradle or cot rather than the bouncer, your arms or at the breast, so he learns that cradle means sleep. Some mothers prefer using the pram for daytime sleeps, as it's convenient to rock wherever you're working.
- With baby on his side, put one of your hands on his shoulder, the other on his bottom, hold him firmly against the mattress, and rhythmically rock his body in a head to toe direction.
- Rapidly jiggle the cradle or cot.
- Soundly pat baby's padded bottom in rhythmical beats about one second apart. Say the word 'shhh' with each beat, leaning close to the baby so he can feel the warmth of your breath.

6 WEEKS

I'd heard about residential parentcraft hospitals from a girlfriend who had been near the end of her tether, and swears it saved her life. I felt now that I needed saving, too — caught in a whirlpool of stress and fatigue, unable to cope with our recurrent settling and posseting problems. My Tresillian day stay nurse booked me in for a week long stay at their Family Care Centre. Tristan had agreed to come as well, and go to work from there each day, so we had a family room with a double bed — and bassinet, of course.

It took me all morning to get organised. What a horrendous task, having to pack a suitcase of baby needs for a week as well as your own gear. In addition to my clothes and toiletries, I'd packed a bag full of baby-care books which I haven't yet found time to read.

We staggered in, just in time for the introductory session after lunch. While the babies were cared for by Tresillian staff, we all sat in a circle with the centre manager (a child health nurse) and discussed why we had come. There was a great deal of empathy as one by one parents spilled out their stories. Everyone else's problems sounded much worse than mine. I felt rather like an imposter. Here I was with a supportive husband, a baby who breastfed heartily and regularly and didn't keep us awake all night, a non-meddlesome family and a good home and income. I made a pledge to count my blessings.

At 6 weeks, Rupert was the youngest baby there, followed by a 9-week-old, then two 17-week babies, who seemed very old (one was even having some solid food). They were all a bit restless in the new environment, maybe catching the air of nervous anticipation from their parents. Rupert was very grizzly, and possetting quite a bit.

Tristan managed to leave work early to get here in time for dinner, which starts at 6 p.m. How wonderful to eat a meal you didn't have to cook (or should I say 'throw together') yourself! Some of the other husbands had come to join in the meal, but I think Tristan was the only one staying the night.

The first evening we were really pampered. In order to give us a good rest the night nurse was to look after the babies in the nursery, bringing them to us when they woke for feeds. After the 7.30 p.m. feed we gratefully handed Rupert over. Tristan stretched out in the family room to watch a bit of TV while I indulged in a long-treasured fantasy — a hot bath, complete with bubbles and a magazine. I could hardly believe my luck, and spent a blissful half hour before retiring to our room. An uninterrupted dinner, relaxed conversation, a long bath, and bed at 8.30 p.m. Certainly a night to remember!

Family care centres

'I have a new baby!' 'I have a life!' These were comments I heard from two women, who had a week earlier spent just a couple of hours at a family care centre, learning the art of settling. Often the problem is not with the baby at all, but it's what we do (or don't do) with them. Some babies don't need much teaching, while others need a good push in the right direction.

If you find that your baby-care practices are not consolidating into a smooth routine by now, or you find yourself often frustrated, depressed (or worse still, violent) then you should consider asking your doctor or child health nurse to refer you to a family care centre — either for a day, or week-long residential stay. You bring along your baby (and partner, too, if he can make it after work). There is usually a long waiting list, so the sooner you make contact the better. Most of the expenses for the week stay are covered by Medicare and your private health fund, if you're in one, although parents pay a small boarding fee.

The wonderful thing about these places (apart from the fact that they save your sanity!) is that you come away feeling that you have a fairly comprehensive knowledge about how to look after your baby; there's not some vital thing you're omitting, or doing the wrong way. And having practical demonstrations, proof that techniques work, is so much better than gaining information via wordy books (even if you do have time to read!). In short, you'll feel more confident and optimistic and, best of all, know that help is at hand if you need it.

6 WEEKS

At Tresillian. Rupert was lying on his back on the bed wailing while I looked on in despair. One of the older nurses, a kind motherly figure, came in response to the sound. She smiled sympathetically at me, then down at the baby. 'What's the matter, little one?' she cooed. Rupert bellowed. She scooped him up, held him level with her face and clicked her tongue, nodding her head up and down. Rupert stopped instantly and stared at her, fascinated. I stared too. What sort of magic was this?

'Distract them', she explained. 'Works every time — unless they're unhappy for a good reason, like hunger or a wet nappy.'

> *It was so simple and effortless. I could actually do something about it. Why hadn't someone told me this before? There's nothing like the advice of a seasoned nurse, who's dealt with every problem and every type of baby.*

A miraculous way to stop crying

All mothers of toddlers know about the art of distraction, but few mothers of newborns have ever heard of it. It's an almost foolproof technique for babies who are at least a few weeks old, and more responsive and alert. It's effective with the sort of crying that continues once you have checked for the obvious causes of discomfort, like hunger, tiredness or a wet nappy, and come up with nothing.

Distraction is commonly practised by child health nurses, but rarely written up in the childcare manuals. It's more easily learnt if demonstrated, so corner someone to show you if you can. Some new mothers use this technique instinctively but to others, caught up in the stress whirlpool and anticipating more complex solutions, it's an eye-opener that something so simple can have such immediate results.

All you do is surprise the baby. Try sweeping him up in your arms, and holding him at face level. Make eye contact, and give a gushing 'Hi there!' in your shrillest voice, accompanied by the most beaming clown-like smile you can muster (open that mouth wide!). With any luck, you'll stop him in his tracks, and he'll look at you with startled eyes, before breaking into an amused grin. The things we do ...!

You can see why this is better demonstrated than described. Of course, there are many variations. You may choose to lean over his face while he's lying on his back. Or produce a (noisy) baby toy. The important things are to make eye contact, and to give your greeting in a sudden burst that will catch his attention and take him off guard. If you can keep exuding your newfound joy — maybe gently waggle him in the air, dance with him, or sing him a song — chances are he'll forget all about torturing you with his crying.

Where does your time go?

At 6 weeks, unable to fathom where my time went, or to explain to my partner why I was still so exhausted, I recorded my movements in detail. Here's a day in the life of a new mum:

3.15–4.15 a.m.	First breastfeed, change, burp, settle.
4.15–4.30 a.m.	Express milk (for work tomorrow).
4.45–7 a.m.	Get some sleep.
7–8.45 a.m.	Second breastfeed, change, play, settle.
8.45–9.15 a.m.	Shower and dress (baby has 30-minute sleep).
9.15–10.15 a.m.	Burp, change, bathe, re-settle.
10.15–10.30 a.m.	Breakfast (baby has 15-minute sleep).
10.30–10.45 a.m.	Soothe and re-settle.
10.45 a.m.–1.30 p.m.	Express milk, work on computer, eat lunch (baby asleep for nearly 3 hours!).
1.30–2.30 p.m.	Third breastfeed (3 large possets).
2.30–3.15 p.m.	Change baby and play.
3.15–3.30 p.m.	Settle baby.
3.30–4.15 p.m.	Washing, phone calls (baby has 45-minute sleep).
4.15–5 p.m.	Baby wakes, change sheets and clothes (extra-large posset), re-settle.
5–7.30 p.m.	Express milk, do dishes.
7.30–8.30 p.m.	Tristan home from work. Breastfeed (baby has $2\frac{1}{2}$ hour sleep).
8.30–10 p.m.	Dinner, play, settle.
10–11 p.m.	Wind down (chat/TV), collapse into bed.

Mind you, this turned out to be quite an abnormal day, in that there were 2 substantial sleeps and only 4 (irregular) feeds. Nevertheless, you can see how difficult it is to find any time for yourself, especially if you want to be diligent and clean up the house as well. Having an office at home, as I did, adds extra pressure, because household and business chores constantly vie for your attention (despite my efforts to keep the professional workload to a minimum).

Late afternoon blues

Late afternoon, or the 'witching hour', is usually the pits for new mums. Baby's unsettled and niggly, you're exhausted and niggly, and you don't know who's influencing who. It can be exacerbated if you have less milk, and baby wants to feed more often.

Try to improve your lot by taking a nap, or at least a rest, as soon as baby goes down in the afternoon (if he goes down!). Forget the housework at this stage! It also helps if you've had a decent breakfast and lunch, rather than running on empty all day. If you're refreshed and fed, you'll be less likely to lose patience with baby and start the cycle off again.

Also consider changes in baby's routine which could help you survive this period. You may both benefit from a late afternoon stroll with the baby pouch or pram, a spell on the baby swing or try baby massage.

7 WEEKS

One of those days. Found myself shaking Rupert's cradle furiously, in a desperate attempt to get him to sleep. Had to make an effort to control myself, catching a scary glimpse of the blinding fury and frustration that take some mothers to the brink. Each time I put him down he would wake half an hour later, crying. I would drop whatever I was doing to rush in and calm him. I didn't know whether he was hungry and needed a top-up feed, tired, in pain, or just plain grumpy. I was spending the whole afternoon either feeding, rocking or patting him on my shoulder.

Finally I remembered the Tresillian technique of controlled settling — after eliminating all obvious causes of crying (like hunger, pain, wet nappy), settle him in the bassinet, leave the room and let him cry for a few minutes before coming back to comfort. I had been loathe to try this (too soft-hearted) but now gave it a go. He was asleep in 3 minutes!

It's hard to do at first, but I guess the experts are right when they say that babies sometimes need to cry for a bit. However, I also agree with the Nursing Mothers' Association decree that 'if he cries for more than a few minutes, he needs you, and the more upset he is the more he needs a loving mother to make everything all right again.'

After lunch I decided to make the effort to take Rupert along to the child health centre for the first session of a postnatal mothers' group which went for 10 weeks. First there was a weigh-in, and Rupert hit the scales at a hefty 6.5 kilograms. Another baby his age weighed only 4.6 kilograms. Rupert's sitting on the 90 per cent line of the graph — meaning he's heavier (and longer) than 90 per cent of babies in his age-group. Takes after his father.

The first session was a chat about our birth experiences. Athough I would have preferred some input on how to handle things now, rather than going back in time, the nurse explained that this topic was always chosen for the first week as many women need to 'get it off their chest'.

It was quite funny to be with women all trying valiantly to control their grumbling, whining, crying, sucking bundles, and hear each other above the din. I wanted to ask some of them how they managed to appear so well groomed, glamorous and at ease, as if they had not a care in the world — while I felt flustered, over-burdened and over-wrought. They must know something I don't!

Baby's checkup

Some mothers like to take baby for one routine postnatal checkup with their hospital paediatrician, as well as checking in with their child health centre. It depends a lot on what your paediatrician suggests while you're in hospital, and whether you have any particular problems. Even though a visit to a paediatrician is not usually necessary, it can be helpful to establish contact, if you can afford the time and money. It means that if your baby has any health problems needing medical attention during the first few months, or indeed, years, you will be able to take baby to a local specialist you already know and like.

The child health centre likes you to check in with them between 6 and 8 weeks. At this second scheduled visit, baby will again be given a thorough physical examination. This time the nurse will be looking in particular at developmental signs, such as smiling, neck strength, interaction. She'll probably chat with you about baby's feeding and sleeping habits, his hearing and vision, the first immunisation and your own well-being and ability to cope. You should also discuss contraception.

Postnatal mothers' groups

Your child health centre or community centre may hold regular weekly group sessions for new mothers, where you bring your baby and chat over coffee for an hour or so, for a period of 6 to 10 weeks. As well as benefiting from the sound practical advice of a health professional, you meet other new mothers at the same stage as yourself. After being cooped up for so long, you'll probably enjoy the chance to get out and relax in a sympathetic environment, where you can feed the baby, check out what your peers are doing, and get some good tips or at least reassurance that you're all in the same boat.

It's best to go along when your baby is only a few weeks old, and you have most to gain. Some centres only take enrolments when babies are 3 months old (but by then your needs are not quite as urgent!).

After the series of sessions has finished, most groups continue to organise their own weekly get-togethers. Many groups have been known to stick together up to pre-school and beyond. Even if you feel that you're too busy or too exhausted to bother with the classes, it's worth making the effort. Long-term bonds like these can prove an invaluable source of comfort through all stages of your baby's growth, not to mention companionship for the babies themselves, and the makings of a trusted baby-sitting club.

Spreading your wings

- Before you go shopping, find out in advance where the good parents' rooms are. Most large department stores in shopping malls have them.
- Consider a baby sling rather than a pram if you want more flexibility (unless your baby is prone to frequent posseting!).
- Catch up with some of the people from your prenatal class. They will probably all have had their babies by now, and could be the makings of a good support group.
- Treat yourself and partner to a restaurant meal. With any luck, baby will sleep right through the meal, comfortably ensconced in a basket at your side (but choose a noisy restaurant, just in case, or a table outside if it's summer).
- Give yourself a real break and get someone to baby-sit — if, by now, you can bear the separation anxiety!
- You could leave the baby with a relative, or in a carefully chosen childcare centre, for a couple of hours each week, in order to give yourself a rest or get a few things done. Don't feel guilty about this — after all, if you're more relaxed, it can only benefit the baby. (See Choosing a childcare centre, pages 185–7.)

Expressing milk

If you're breastfeeding, child minding or baby-sitting usually presents the extra burden of providing breastmilk for the feeds you miss unless you're in the fortunate position of being able to slip over to the centre at the appropriate time, and feed him yourself.

Some women may be going back to work, either full or part time. If this is the case, they may choose to combine breastfeeding (morning and evening), with formula given by the carer during the day. This

1 MONTH OLD (4–7 WEEKS)

usually means expressing milk during the day for breast health, whether or not you choose to keep and store the milk.

For those who have to spend time away from their babies, but want to continue feeding them breastmilk, it's important to have a full knowledge of the art and hygiene of expressing milk.

Expressing tips

- Use a one-handed battery-operated or electric pump; with your free hand, you can help the milk flow by massaging the breast towards the nipple.

- If you're having difficulty, try a different position. For example, sit with your knees bent and legs apart, leaning forward so that your arms rest on your thighs and breasts hang down in between. It's not elegant, but helps the milk flow freely.

- Thinking of baby encourages let down. You could also focus on his photo.

- If your breasts are very full or hard, you could take the opportunity to express a little milk from each before you feed. Always supplement this foremilk with some of the richer hindmilk, expressed after the baby has fed.

- Unless you already have a supply frozen, you'll need to think ahead and express a little surplus milk after each feed for a few days before, so you have the required amount all bottled and ready for the baby-sitter.

- If you need breastmilk for the following day, the night or early morning is a good time to express. Usually your breasts are full, and the baby doesn't take as much milk as during the day. But it means losing valuable sleep while you stay up expressing, not to mention the pressure of meeting your volume requirements. Another disadvantage of the last-minute rush is that expressing large amounts of milk will increase your milk supply, which is exactly what you don't need when you're going out without the baby.

> • To get maximum milk supply in one sitting, feed baby one breast (or more if he needs it) at the first morning feed, and fully express the other. If you have a one-handed pump, you can do this simultaneously.

Expressing while away from home

When you're away from the baby for more than a few hours, your breasts will tell you when it's feeding time — and you'll need to express milk, if at all possible. If you leave it for too long, they could turn into hard, painful melons.

This means packing your handbag or briefcase with the required equipment: breast pump (if you use one), hand towel to protect your clothing and mop up the drips, an empty sterile bottle and insulated bag pre-packed with ice or freezer packs. After all, you don't want to painstakingly express all that precious milk only to pour it down the sink (as many of us have had to do when travelling unprepared).

People talk blithely about expressing breastmilk, but never go into detail about just where you're going to do it when you're out, or how difficult or time-consuming it can be compared with your baby's competent sucking. You might be relegated to the unsanitary confines of a toilet, the back of a car, or someone's office (usually uncurtained). You may see other mothers breastfeeding in public, but how many do you see breast pumping? It's not exactly socially acceptable and not always a pretty sight! Furthermore, you're inevitably under pressure when you're expressing milk away from home. You may be insecure about the environment, or have only 15 minutes in which to complete the task. Or you may be dripping milk all over your best suit or evening dress.

Stress, of course, makes expressing more difficult and time consuming, so it's a vicious circle. You just have to try to switch off, relax, and think 'baby thoughts' to get your milk flowing. It's important to express until there are no hard lumps, to avoid the risk of mastitis (see pages 79–80).

Tips for storing expressed milk

- You can store breastmilk in the centre-back of the fridge for 3–5 days (formerly 48 hours); in the freezer compartment of the fridge for 2 weeks; in a separate freezer of a 2-door fridge for 3 months; in a deep freezer for 6–12 months. Use special plastic bags for freezing small amounts or freeze in a sterile ice-cube tray.

- Label each bottle or bag with the date and amount.

- When filling bottles in stages, never add freshly expressed milk to frozen milk, as this thaws out the top layer. Cool it in the fridge first, and then add it to the frozen bottle.

- Keep some milk frozen in lots of about 50 ml for baby-sitters. They can use this for a top-up or soother if required, rather than having to defrost a whole bottle, and then throw most of it away.

- Thaw in the fridge. Milk thawed in this way will last for 24 hours in the fridge. Or thaw quickly, by holding the frozen bottle or bag under warm running water. (Don't microwave, as this may destroy some of the nutrients.) Milk thawed this way should only be kept 4 hours.

- Never refreeze thawed milk, just as you never refreeze any frozen foods. Discard any milk left over after feeding.

Sleeping through

Depending on how frequently your baby feeds, this may simply mean dropping one feed during the night, so that baby sleeps from last feed in the evening (say 10 p.m.) until the early morning (around 4–5 a.m.), skipping the 1–2 a.m. wake-up call.

For some fortunate parents, this happens by about 7 weeks. For us, it occurred only once at 7 weeks but still, it was a delightful glimpse of what was to come! So if this happens to you, try not to get too excited. It could well be a false alarm and your cunning baby may then wait several more weeks before again delighting you with his deep sleep abilities. At least now you know he's capable of the feat.

Other babies will trick you by dropping the 10.30 p.m. feed, instead of the 1–2 a.m. feed, so that you have to go to bed really early to take advantage of the precious 5-hour stretch of sleep (which may be difficult if your partner doesn't come home till late). You could try waking him for the 10.30 p.m. feed, to coax a change in his pattern, but you'll probably find he's sleeping too deeply to wake. (See Sleep patterns, pages 179–80.)

If your baby refuses to drop a feed, he's not abnormal: many mothers find themselves still getting up to feed once or twice a night until at least the 3-month mark. You may like to encourage him by shortening the night feeds. Some mothers try giving water instead.

Growth spurts

If you're weighing your baby every week, you'll probably be delighted at the proof of progress. ('400 grams in one week!' I heard one mother of a 5-week-old exclaim with pride. 'No wonder my arms are aching!') But something a lot of mothers don't realise is that baby may have spurts of growth at various stages in development, resulting in sudden appetite increases. This could happen at approximately 3 to 4 weeks, 6 weeks and 12 weeks, although it varies considerably.

If you find your baby is crying without apparent cause, or waking earlier than usual, it may simply mean that he is hungry again, and for a time needs more frequent feeding. It's important to be aware of this possibility, otherwise you may try in vain to re-settle the baby, mistaking his cries for tiredness.

Looking after your body

• Don't neglect your back (by now overburdened with breastfeeding, baby capsules and bending over). Tummy exercises will help strengthen back muscles.

• Use the correct posture to pick up and carry heavy loads, by bending your knees and taking the weight on your thighs, not your back.

• Remember your pelvic floor exercises — a nuisance, but they should be done to avoid the risk of saggy muscles leading to incontinence (and to improve your sex life).

• Try to find the time and energy to put on a fitness videotape, or jump on an exercise cycle for a short time every day.

• If you can go to the gym, you'll find that most have a creche, open for daytime sessions.

• Get enough rest, eat well, and take care breasts do not become swollen or hard.

A father's view

The first 6 weeks are pretty tough. Having made it this far, there are many intriguing developments this month as your child becomes more aware and a little more active.

Family care centres are life savers

For many first timers, this is also the period when the exhaustion and intensity of looking after the baby can go beyond your resources and resolve. Professional help may be needed.

If a live-in session at a family care centre is advised, don't let your partner go alone. It is essential that you join in. You really do have everything to learn from these wonderful teachers. In a few days you will pick up fantastic techniques to alleviate crying, reflux and mutual exhaustion, and develop ways to maximise your baby's sleep. It is not a 'women's-only' domain, and it's more than likely you will come out a better man. Family care centres are not five star hotels, but stick it out if you can.

Breastmilk in your tea?

By now the larder will be well and truly bare, and you may be considering Red Cross parcels and handouts from neighbours (if they still visit). This is perfectly natural, and a good way to lose weight. But mark my words, you will get to the day (or night) when after 20 hours of exhaustion and a baby that is gently screaming itself to sleep you want nothing in the world more than a cup of tea.

You scrape the last of the tea into the pot and, despite thinking you ran out of milk yesterday, you discover a small amount in a plastic jug way down the back of the fridge. True, it does make what appears to be a cup of tea, but it will not be something you admit to, or repeat too often. Although your partner will wonder why the 50 ml of expressed milk evaporated to just 20 ml, you will remain silent. They are right, breastmilk is for babies.

The first smile
It is usually around this time that (often for no apparent reason) your baby will look you in the eye and give you the most amazing toothless smile. If it's the first, like it was for me, don't gloat too much, as your partner will be crushed that her 20 hours a day of contact has not reaped the reward. The anticipation of the next one will calm the waters.

Five top games fathers can play with their babies
Just because your baby seems only to sleep, cry and feed, doesn't mean you can't play some delightful games together. Football, trampolines and bungee jumping will have to come later. What you can do right now is start the communication process and have a great deal of fun while you're at it. Add these to your favourites:

Holding hands
Babies have an amazingly strong grip. Daddy's little finger is the perfect size. Jiggling or just holding it is a great way to make contact. Some babies, however, just don't want to let go — so don't try this if you are in a hurry to go somewhere. He may also assume it's a very long nipple and immediately put it to his mouth.

Bath time
Most babies have a great affinity with water. This is a great time for some soothing words and gentle contact. Remember to keep his head supported and test the water temperature first. Bath time can be such fun.

Three in a bed
Bed is a great place to have a chat, make silly noises or just catch up on sleep. You'll find yourself gazing for hours or just playing and napping. This is a relaxing way to share some great moments.

Peek-a-boo
A perennial favourite. Peek-a-boo is, I think, the ultimate silly game that all babies love. Try to do it gently, as babies can often be startled by sudden movements. This just may, in the weeks ahead, give you the first smile.

Daddy dancing
Rhythmic movements are another great distraction. Swaying or bouncing to music can be a magical way to transform cry-baby into perfect-baby. Just remember to keep the baby well supported and to make all movements gentle.

Daddy talk

It's never too soon to tell your child about football competitions, television programs and news from the office. It's the intimacy, animation and warmth of your voice that your baby finds interesting, not so much the content.

A natural extension to this is singing — a sure-fire winner, and great relaxant for fathers and babies alike. Fortunately babies are totally non-judgmental and will enjoy everything that comes out of your mouth, no matter how tuneless. A great confidence booster. (Another father I know explained the difference — in great detail — between the Senate and the House of Representatives, simply because he couldn't think of anything else to say. He tells me the baby was enthralled throughout, hanging on every word.)

2 MONTHS OLD (8–11 WEEKS)

MILESTONES

- Lots of baby talk.
- Lots of smiles, chuckles and gurgles.
- Raises head to watch things while on tummy.
- Develops good head control.
- Discovers own hands and legs.
- May stop crying if spoken to.
- Turns at the sound of your voice.
- Follows you with his eyes.
- May reach out to touch things (involuntary reflex).
- May sleep through the night by the end of the month.

WHAT THEY NEVER TELL YOU THIS MONTH

- Baby should have 5–10 minutes of tummy time between daytime feeds.
- Baby should have a good sleep between each feed.
- Put baby to bed as soon as he displays signs of tiredness.
- Possetting and reflux are different things.

THINGS TO DO THIS MONTH

- First round of immunisation (8 weeks).
- Child health centre checkup (8 weeks).
- Buy a cot (if you haven't one already).
- Have some fun with baby.

CHAPTER SIX

2 months old (8–11 weeks)

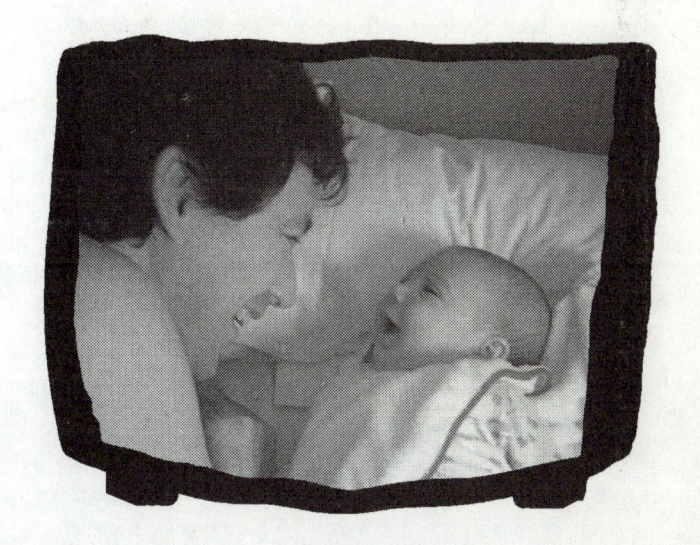

8 WEEKS

What a wonderful feeling, to go to your baby in the morning when he stirs, lean over his bassinet to say hello, and be rewarded with a big smile which lights up his sleepy face. And to think that just a few weeks ago I was worried that my little baby might not warm to me, frightened he might associate me with discomfort because he cried so often in my arms, and was oblivious to my frustrated attempts to solve his problems.

At last we feel he is getting to know us. He will now usually turn at the sound of our voices. And the sight of his deep green almond-shaped eyes staring intently up at me while I'm breastfeeding is heart-melting.

He's starting to consistently recognise other things, too. The last few mornings when I've placed him on the change table, he's looked up at his colourful musical clowns dangling overhead, and his face has broken into a delighted grin.

Your baby this month

This month your baby will do a lot of smiling. Previously, you may have had to 'earn' your smiles, but now they'll be given in abundance, along with chuckles and lots of baby talk. His rapid development is exciting to watch. He'll start to clutch his bib, or your clothing. He'll reach out and touch your face, or try to grasp dangling rattles and other objects which catch his attention. He'll turn at the sound of your voice, and later his eyes will follow you around the room. He'll recognise other people who are close to him. He'll be very interested in his environment (including television and videos). By the end of the month he may use his arms to lift up the top half of his body when placed on his tummy. You'll find he moves around his cradle or cot. And then there's play. Suddenly you'll find that he's awake for so much longer — and you have to find ways of amusing him! He will probably graduate from cradle to cot this month, if he hasn't already.

8 WEEKS

Watching Tristan and Rupert together this morning was so touching. After the morning breastfeed in bed I heaved open the curtains to let the sunshine in, and went to make a cup of tea. When I returned I found them face to face on the pillow, Tristan making earnest conversation while tiny Rupert gazed at him with rapt attention, lips curved in a smile, occasionally making little noises of acknowledgment or chuckles of joy, chubby pink legs waving wildly in the air. What a father–son rapport. Tristan's so playful with him, and is always thinking up new games to make him laugh. This as well as being a whiz at nappy changing and having a bottomless pit of tenderness and patience to walk the floor with Rupert during the bad times. I really am so lucky to have him as a husband and father.

Handling baby

There's no longer any need to handle baby with kid gloves. Fathers can now hold baby up in the air and get away with it! But no heavy jolting or shaking. By 8 weeks you shouldn't have to support his head any more, except when lying him down. Baby should now be doing most of the work himself. Offer him a wide variety of positions. For example, try carrying him in a sideways position, so he can see what's going on around him.

Visual stimulation

Help baby's eyesight to develop by providing lots of visual interest, in the form of mobiles, soft toys and strong colours. Two-month-old babies prefer round shapes to geometric shapes, and patterned textures to plain. The 'black-and-white' phase has passed, and bright colours, rather than contrasts, are now the go. How about some big red smiles?

Extended tummy time

By the beginning of this month, baby should be having at least 5–10 minutes of floor time on his tummy between feeds. You judge the best time: some babies posset if you put them down on their tummy straight after a feed. Try to increase this time daily, until he's spending more time face down than face up. As he gets stronger, and is able to lift his head higher and sustain it for longer periods, he'll gain more enjoyment from being able to look about the room. Your baby may be pushing up on his arms already, although some won't do this until next month. Make sure there are some interesting toys (or a mirror) close enough to catch his attention.

As well as floor play, give your baby tummy time in other situations, such as carrying him face down, or having him lie on top of you in bed or in the bath. (See also Tummy time, pages 129–30.)

Routine versus spontaneity

As you meet more mothers, you'll probably find there are two schools of thought: those who religiously follow a strict routine with baby, which takes priority over all else, and those who carry on regardless, making baby fit in with their plans.

Mothers in the first category wait until baby wakes up before leaving the house, unwilling to risk waking him before his time, aware that if baby misses, say, the morning sleep, they will spend the rest of the day paying for it. Their life and appointments are dictated by the baby's sleeping and feeding patterns.

Mothers in the second group will whisk up a sleeping baby and transfer him to the pram or car, unconcerned if he wakes in the process (although often he doesn't). They may feed when the baby wakes, or may wait until he cries. They roll along happily, while the baby seems to fit in just as happily.

Whichever category you fit into is probably dictated to some extent by your personality, by what you've been taught, and to a large extent by your baby — whether he's a good sleeper, a light sleeper, difficult to settle, and so on. The point is, don't find yourself feeling insecure or incompetent because another mother's way works best for her.

8 WEEKS

What hits you, if you're not used to it, is the incredible sameness of the days. You wake up in the morning (at an ungodly hour) and you're so tired, but the feed has to go on. You know that after an hour or two you'll be able to put him to sleep (hopefully), and snatch some time to shower, have breakfast, do a few chores. Then it'll be feed, burp, change, feed, sleep and settle (or walk the floor).

> *Sure, you can liven things up if you so desire (if you're organised or awake enough!) by taking baby out for a walk or to visit friends, but you can't alter the basic routine. And that's probably the biggest change to my life, having been used to doing things spontaneously. A routine of any sort has become foreign. And yet now a tiny tyrant is imposing one upon me.*
>
> *Not that I'm complaining about having a tiny tyrant — he's still the most wonderful thing that ever happened to us!*

A word to working women

If you've been working up until having the baby, and especially if you've had this baby later in life, then you're liable to be even harder hit by the chaos this little being generates. You're used to being organised, efficient, on schedule, *in charge*. And suddenly, you're out of control! It's a difficult adjustment, and unless you have a model baby, you're liable to become frustrated and depressed, and see yourself as a failure.

You were going to be the exception — the one who always looked well groomed and attractive, had the house shining and clean, the baby gurgling happily, the business side under control, and greeted your man at the end of the afternoon with a serene demeanour and a cheery smile (complete with lipstick)!

It can be bewildering and disheartening to find yourself spending all day in a tracksuit, seemingly not achieving anything of substance. To miss sleep, miss meals and feel like a wreck. To have the house continually in a mess and to resort too often to takeaway meals. To be in a public place with your child screaming his lungs out, and feel humiliated but helpless to quieten his cries.

This may not be you. But if it is, try not to be too hard on yourself. Don't feel it's your fault, or that you're incompetent. You have to change your perspective, to focus on all that you're giving to, and gaining from, your new baby.

Breast pads

Some women find they don't need these, others wear them regularly. As with nappies, you have a choice of disposable or washable. (Washable may be better if you have sore nipples.) It's advisable to wear them while out — you just never know when a 'baby thought' will start the flow. I've heard some woeful stories from working girlfriends. One was sitting in a meeting when she (and others) suddenly became aware of two rapidly spreading milk stains on her silk shirt; another woman was catching up with old workmates at a luncheon, and had to dash from the table to mop up. Never were faces so red!

8 WEEKS

Finally caught up with my obstetrician for a checkup, 2 weeks late. There was a half-hour wait, so I carried Rupert in his capsule to the coffee shop downstairs. I'd missed breakfast as usual, so a cappuccino and a sandwich were much in need.

The second the steaming cup touched the table Rupert let out a wail, and it continued unabated. People looked up from magazines and tete-a-tetes. I gritted my teeth in embarrassment and hissed at Rupert to be quiet. I tried every trick in the book but he was determined to make a spectacle of us.

Grimly, I picked up my coffee and the capsule, and headed for a table in the corner where we weren't so conspicuous (and hopefully were more out of earshot). The waitress trotted after me with the untouched sandwich. By now I was starving, and just dying for a hot drink. I jiggled the capsule and pleaded with him to hush. He took a deep breath and turned up the volume.

Totally humiliated and feeling as if all eyes in the restaurant were upon me, I accepted defeat. Leaving the coveted snack on the table, I scooped up baby and bags, and high-tailed it back to the consulting room, where the wailing suddenly and mysteriously stopped. Life can be cruel.

Immunisation

Triple antigen is a 'three-in-one' vaccine for protection against diphtheria, tetanus and whooping cough. It's given in conjunction with oral Sabin (against polio) and the relatively new vaccination Hib (Haemophilus influenzae, type b), which has nothing to do with the 'flu, but is a major cause of many life-threatening diseases in children under 5. The first triple antigen is due at 2 months, with follow ups at 4 and 6 months, and boosters later on.

Occasionally babies have adverse reactions, such as high temperatures; more often they just become flushed and a bit grizzly. As well as the injection, there's the bruised swelling from the needle. Have some infant paracetamol at hand just in case. (The Health Department suggests giving paracetamol half an hour before the injection, but I prefer only using drugs when proven necessary.) Your baby may sleep longer than usual after the event, which is okay. Only in rare cases are there more serious complications.

Although strongly recommended by health authorities, immunisation is a controversial issue. If you have any doubts, seek as much information as you can from a variety of sources to put your mind at rest.

Get outdoors

When you're feeling cooped up, the baby's crying, or you've run out of ways to entertain him, don't underestimate the wonder of nature. Just to lay a rug out on the grass, in your backyard or a nearby park, gives both you and your baby a break. He can feel the wind on his face and watch butterflies and trees move, while you may even have the chance to read the newspapers or a magazine. Or put him in the baby sling or pram and go for a walk. You may find your crying baby becomes wondrously serene as he gazes about with eyes wide. And all that stimulation and fresh air seems to work magic with settling him later on.

Help in your own home

Many women don't realise that home visits by specialist helpers may well be an option, depending on where you live. You might feel the need for a mothercraft nurse to help with settling, or a lactation consultant to help with feeding difficulties. Apart from the blissful convenience of having someone come to you, it can be more effective and confidence boosting to have your problems looked at in your own environment. After all, if someone else can stop the crying or put baby to sleep in his own familiar surroundings, then you should be able to mimic those actions and achieve the same results. (Well, that's the general idea.)

8 WEEKS

A wearing week it's been. I'm concerned about Rupert's daytime sleep 'pattern' (too often he's sleeping in 30–45 minute bursts, rather than a solid 2-hour sleep) and about his continued frequent posseting. Tristan and I still walk around with towels permanently draped over our shoulders to catch the spills. Today, anguished and exhausted, I rang Tresillian again. They have a service called Outreach (which fortunately operates in our area), where a child health nurse comes out to your home for a couple of hours, free of charge, to help sort out your problems with the baby. It's wonderful, because they can see first-hand what happens in your home, and give you survival techniques which you can practise under supervision on your own turf.

What if baby only sleeps for 45 minutes?

If you settle the baby after a feed, only to find him waking 30–45 minutes later, you should try to re-settle, rather than just get him up. He really needs to sleep for another hour or two. You may think that sleeping for only short periods during the day will help him sleep longer at night but, in fact it may have the reverse effect, making him overtired, and so thwarting good sleep at night. It's said that sleep engenders sleep. Get them into the habit, and they'll sleep better and longer!

Waking at short intervals is a fairly common occurrence during the first few months, as baby's natural sleep pattern is in 45–50 minute cycles, comprising a light, dreaming sleep (or 'rapid eye movement' phase), followed by a period of a deeper sleep (this reverses at 3 months). Babies have a tendency to wake up between phases or cycles. They need coaxing back to sleep, to learn to sleep longer.

Try leaving him to cry on his own for a few minutes if he wakes, rather than dashing straight in to see what's wrong. Often this will be enough to send him back to sleep. If this doesn't work, go in and try your usual settling techniques. Don't pick baby up at this stage unless it's obviously a wet or dirty nappy, in which case a quick change may be all he needs to drift off again.

9 WEEKS

I've realised I have to change my perspective, in order to enjoy quality time with the baby. How awful to have regrets later on about lost opportunities! I've been trying to get too many things done during the day — which means I often try to squeeze in phone calls or chores, while the baby's preoccupied with his rattle or gurgling in his cot. This should stop! I see now that every moment of his waking time is precious, as he's developing so quickly and, besides, he needs my full presence. I'm sure he senses it when my attention is elsewhere.

Often a cry during waking time is simply a call for attention, which ceases as soon as he's picked up or even spoken to. It makes you realise that what you thought was a tragic cry of real pain and despair maybe wasn't so bad after all.

Have some fun with baby

One theory is that the baby's moods are often set by the mother. If she's tense, uncertain or depressed, the baby will react to that. If she's relaxed, happy and positive, the baby will respond. If this is true, you could find yourself trapped in a vicious circle: your stress leads to an unsettled baby, leading to more stress.

So learn to relax. Lighten up, and enjoy your baby. This is one lesson I wish someone had drummed into me. Get into the habit of stopping everything from time to time and putting your worries aside, even if just for a couple of minutes. Close your eyes, take a few deep breaths, and centre yourself. Give baby a tickle, shake a rattle, or make up a game to play. For example, you could lie down on your back with legs bent, put baby on your legs with his hands on your knees, and pull him towards you. Or hold him on your lap, pull him up by his hands, and support him while he has a kick or jig. Enjoy his enjoyment. You and the baby will both benefit.

Baby amusements

- Music box with pull string (hung out of reach), or wind-up musical mobile.
- Battery-operated or wind-up toys that move or make noises.
- Soft washable toys.
- Rattles and squeaky toys.
- Introduce baby to a toy frame, or activity gym. Great for tummy time, as well as time on his back and in his portable chair.
- Position or hang toys and rattles close to baby's face, so he'll be able to reach out and touch them with ease. His eyes are focusing only up to his own arm length, so colourful blurry shapes out of his reach may only frustrate him.

9 WEEKS

Tristan and I bought a cot and had great fun setting it up in his nursery, together with a baby monitor. The cot has a brightly patterned quilt and a vivid red bumper (which fits around the inside to prevent him bumping his head or trapping his arm between the railings). No pillow at this age, of course, but because Rupert possets so much we've laid an absorbent nappy, covered by a pillowcase, where he rests his head. Last night we spent the evening hanging assorted mobiles above the cot at various heights, to provide him with lots of visual stimulation.

Up until yesterday, he'd only slept in it during the day — he looked so tiny and unprotected on the vast mattress that we worried he might feel insecure, and wanted to introduce him gradually to the experience. But last night we planned the big move — from sharing our bedroom in his bassinet, to a room of his own. It felt like the first day at school — such a wrench. What a big boy, sleeping in a cot. After having him in a cradle by our bed for so long, I really missed him during the night. He went to sleep huddled in one corner, against the bumper, with teddy bears for company. As for me, I woke regularly throughout the night to go and check on him. So much for getting more sleep!

From cradle to cot

Depending on your baby's size and mobility, you will probably want to move him from his bassinet to a cot in the next month or two, if you haven't already done so. He may start looking a little squashed, or move in his sleep and hit the side of the bassinet, waking himself up. If he's been sleeping in your bedroom up until now, this is a logical time to move him to a separate room as cots do tend to take up a lot of space! You may have been using the nursery just for changing and storage but now it can bloom as a functioning part of the house. It can be a big step, giving baby a room of his own.

9 WEEKS

We never did get a repeat performance of Rupert sleeping through the night. Wonder when he'll drop the 2 a.m. feed for good? It would be a treat to sleep through until 5 a.m. I remember before we had the baby I used to wonder how parents could bear to be woken so early by their children (by that I meant 7.30 a.m.!); and how they could sacrifice the luxury (dare I say necessity) of a sleep-in at weekends. That would be a major drawback, I thought.

Now it's the least of my worries. I don't think of complaining (most of the time), because the pull towards that little body who needs me is so great, it swamps everything else. The hour I'm roused doesn't matter — although getting enough sleep, in total, is certainly a concern. Six hours straight would be bliss!

Feeding quantities

Many mothers who give bottles are unsure whether or not they're overfeeding their baby. Depending on baby's size and appetite, amongst other things, an average bottlefeed for a 9-week-old can range from around 150 ml to 210 ml. Work out the approximate quantity needed for each feed by multiplying your baby's weight by 150, and dividing by the number of feeds per day.

For example: 7 kilograms x 150 = 1050 ml (intake per day), divided by 5 feeds = approximately 210 ml per feed. Remember, though, that babies don't necessarily take the same quantity at each feed — it's the amount consumed per day that's more important (about 150 ml for each kilogram of baby's ideal body weight).

Although you can overfeed your baby with formula, it's often said that 'you can't overfeed a breastfed baby', although no-one has been able to satisfactorily explain to me why this is the case. Also, it's not a belief shared by all the experts. A lactation consultant told me that you could certainly overfeed when breastfeeding, particularly if you have a baby with a strong sucking tendency, which may be mistaken for hunger. Instead of putting him back on the empty breast to suck, his mother may put him on the full one, giving him lots of milk he doesn't really want or need.

Breast comfort

By now most breastfeeding mothers find their breasts no longer feel continually swollen or bloated. You may wonder where your milk has gone. The happy news is that there is still plenty of milk, only the discomfort has disappeared. Some women (not me, I hasten to add) choose this time to substitute a bottle of formula for a breastfeed during the day, either to give themselves more flexibility (by being able to stay out for the afternoon and leave baby with a sitter) or give themselves a break at home while their partner takes over the feeding. Although this may be frowned upon by lactation experts, at least it's not considered as big a sin as introducing formula during the vital first 6 weeks.

(See Combining bottle and breast, page 197.)

10 WEEKS

This morning while breastfeeding I looked down at Rupert, said hello and smiled. To my surprise, he loosened his grip on the breast (normally ferociously secure) and gave me a big smile back! I laughed delightedly, and kept talking, and Rupert seemed to lapse into a fit of the giggles, grinning and chuckling in between sucks. I finally had to take him off the breast for a minute and have a chat with him, before resuming feeding in a more sober fashion! How lovely — he's never been like this before.

But the most dramatic progress this week has been in the hands department. He seems to be aware of them at last. The once clenched little fists are now more relaxed and open, and he's clasping them together often, in sleep and waking mode. Tonight in bed Tristan held up his finger, wiggling it close to Rupert's chin, and Rupert grasped it (after a few hit and misses). This was then repeated many times, with us an appreciative and enthralled audience.

How quickly he's progressing now. There was another 'first' when I placed him in his portable chair to examine his dangling rattles. After staring at them intently for some time, he swung his hand vigorously and banged one, over and over again. It lurched backwards and forwards with a vengeance, almost hitting him full on the nose. (I had to catch it once or twice in case it hurt him.) I watched in fascination as he continued this game for some minutes.

His attention span in the chair is getting much longer. In the early days he would stay there for only a couple of minutes before starting to whinge. Now he's content for 10 minutes or more.

Hands and legs

Around the 10-week mark you'll be delighted to find baby's hands starting to become functional, as he begins to discover how they work — although at this stage, much of the clutching movement is still an involuntary reflex. Over the next few weeks, he may spend lots of time studying his hands, an endless source of fascination and amusement and, at this stage, the best toys he's got. Help baby to explore and find out his capabilities. Try tickling his palm.

Over the next few weeks you'll also notice more activity in the legs department. Help baby develop by giving him as much time as possible without his nappy, both on his back and on his tummy, so he can move his legs about in complete freedom. (Find an absorbent underlay or quilt for baby to lie on, one which you can throw in the wash.) You can even buy socks with rattles on them, to add to his enjoyment.

11 WEEKS

I've been taking Rupert into the big bath with me for several weeks now. He hardly fits in the basin these days. It's a lovely relaxing time for us, lying back in the deep warm water with his slippery naked body against mine.

He always enjoys his baths, smiling and chuckling, but this afternoon he went quite crazy. I was supporting him in floating position on his back, when he suddenly started kicking his legs frantically, squealing with delight at the big splash they made. His plump little legs kept thrashing in wild abandon, while I marvelled at his energy and staying power. He went non-stop for several minutes, revelling in every second of his new-found mobility.

What happened to the sedate little creature who used to lay passively on my arm? Baths will never be the same again.

Big baths and showers

Sharing the big bath with baby has many advantages: it's fun, it's relaxing for both of you, it's nice and deep for baby and there's plenty of opportunity for kicking and splashing. When filling the bath, remember to run cold water last, so the metal of the hot tap doesn't burn him. And don't have the bath water quite as hot as you would normally (if in doubt, buy a baby bath temperature gauge).

A bath ring with suction feet is useful to keep baby safe and contained when he's at the sitting-up stage. Or you could use a rubber mat to help avoid slipping.

You may like to take baby into the shower with you (dads often snap up this job). The warm running water seems to have a soothing effect, and most babies enjoy it. But beware — babies can be like slippery eels; take care he doesn't slide through your arms onto the hard tiles.

11 WEEKS

I'm becoming so distressed with Rupert's constant posseting that I decided to seek further help. Some people have suggested it's reflux and needs medication, others say not to worry. The trouble is, you really need to spend time with the baby and observe his behaviour before passing judgment. I obtained a referral to a local day stay run by a hospital and community health service.

In charge of the centre was Kath, an experienced child health nurse, sensible and down-to-earth. We sat in the cosy family room and chatted while I fed Rupert. Occasionally you come across a real gem like Kath. I found her ideas and methods more practical and logical to my mind than most of the information in the books I'd consulted. She just made sense.

For instance, some people say posseting is due to overfeeding — an overflow from a full stomach — which puts you in a dilemma about how long to leave the baby at the breast. But Kath said that overfeeding wasn't always the cause: 'You can see it's not the case with Rupert — at this feed anyway — because he's eager to feed again, even though he's posseted after the first breast.' She smiled reassuringly. 'It's just immature plumbing, a leaky valve which will soon fix itself. Nothing to worry about!' Kath was the first person to explain this to me. If she's right, refusing him more milk would leave me with an irritable baby and not necessarily stop the posseting.

Kath said that when I put Rupert down I should allow him to cry for 5 minutes or so to help him learn how to settle himself, which I've started to do anyway. Also, rather than going in immediately to comfort him if he continues to cry, she suggested I wait for a lull, then whip in to pat, jiggle or stroke him. That way he won't think that putting on a show of hysteria is an effective way to summon a parent.

But her best tip was not to put him down according to the clock. (I'd previously been told to put him down 1½ hours after a feed.) Instead, react to the sometimes subtle signs of tiredness, such as grizzling, pulling a face or clenching his hands. It might even happen straight after a feed. 'If he's crying or unhappy,' Kath said, 'it almost certainly means bedtime.'

What a revelation! How many times had we paced the floor for hours, trying to quiet our crying baby, thinking it may be wind, colic or reflux, when it may have been fatigue?

Of course, at the centre today Rupert showed no signs of any discomfort. He went to sleep like an angel, slept most of the day and hardly posseted at all after feeds. Why do they do this to us?

Posseting or reflux?

These conditions are not, as some people think, synonymous. There is harmless posseting (spilling of milk), and there is reflux, where the baby obviously has some discomfort (and the milk does not necessarily come up through the mouth). The two conditions are often confused, and the more you investigate, the more confused you're likely to get, due to various professionals using the same word to mean different things.

The confusion lies in the fact that 'reflux' is officially an umbrella term, meaning any leaking of the stomach contents (milk or stomach

2 MONTHS OLD (8-11 WEEKS)

acid) into the lower oesophagus — whether or not it actually comes all the way up through the mouth. But most people use this term to refer specifically to the more serious type of reflux, where stomach acid is involved. To make the distinction clearer, here is a more detailed definition of the two conditions.

Posseting
This simply means bringing up milk after a feed. It may also be referred to as regurgitation or vomiting.

About 50 per cent of babies posset, due to an immature or weak valve between the stomach and oesophagus which allows the milk to escape and flow back up. In most babies it is a perfectly normal physiological process without complications, causing no pain or discomfort. It usually settles at around 3 months, when they start to sit up (which strengthens the valve), or at least by 7 to 9 months, when they're well into solids.

However you may still find it upsetting if your baby possets a lot, and worry that he's not getting enough milk. On top of that, there's the mess, smell and possible embarrassment. Some experts advise giving the baby a powder which you mix with breastmilk, to thicken the contents of his stomach and help keep the milk down. However, it's expensive, hard to administer (by teaspoon) and often doesn't work anyway. If baby is happy, alert and putting on weight, it's best simply to put up with the inconvenience. Get used to wearing a nappy or towel over your shoulder and doing extra loads of washing, and wait until he grows out of it.

Dealing with posseting
- Sit baby up in a portable chair for 10–15 minutes after feeding.
- Put a small pillow under his mattress, to raise the head of his bed when he sleeps.
- Cut bunny rugs into four, to use in the cot under baby's head for milk spillage. Or use a nappy, with a folded sheet on top for softness.

Reflux

(This may be referred to as gastric reflux, oesophageal reflux or, officially, gastro-oesophageal reflux.)

Unlike posseting, reflux *does* cause the baby discomfort and there is usually disruption of feeding and maybe sleeping patterns. Baby may cry during or after feeding. He may pull off the breast, arch his back, become rigid, writhe, kick or throw out his arms. Reflux is similar to adult heartburn — a discomfort or burning sensation due to stomach acids leaking back into the baby's sensitive oesophagus, along with the milk. This leakage can lead to inflammation and poor weight gain (even loss of weight), along with constant crying and irritability. If this is the case, your baby needs prompt medical attention.

The condition can be difficult to diagnose because a baby with reflux doesn't necessarily bring milk up through the mouth. Your doctor may prescribe an antacid mixture to give him after feeding, to see if this settles him. Or a powder which mixes to a gluggy paste, and also contains antacid (not popular with some doctors, because it can lead to constipation, and contains salt or sodium which may overload the baby's system). There's another medication which helps to empty the contents of the stomach faster.

As frustrating as it is for the parent, it seems just a case of 'try it and see'. If one of these medications does the trick, then reflux was most probably the cause of his crying.

It's worth checking with your child health nurse to see whether there is a Vomiting Infants Support Association in your area.

Dealing with reflux

- Any treatment should first be discussed with your doctor.

- Keep the head end of baby's mattress propped up, using a pillow, rolled towel or phone books underneath. If this makes his bassinet or cot dangerously shallow, try bricks under the legs of the bassinet instead.

- Lay an adult pillow under baby's head and shoulders on the changing table.

2 MONTHS OLD (8–11 WEEKS)

- Change before a feed.
- Wipe his bottom by turning baby sideways, rather than pulling legs up to the tummy (which may force stomach acid into the oesophagus).
- After feeding, sit baby semi-upright in a portable chair for 15 minutes, to help settle the milk.
- Some experts suggest avoiding substances like caffeine (in tea, coffee and chocolate), alcohol and nicotine, claiming these affect baby through your breastmilk by weakening pressure in his tummy valve. However this is not generally accepted.

11 WEEKS

The day we've been waiting for, ever since that false alarm one month ago at 7 weeks — Rupert finally slept through the night! And he did it magnificently, going down like a model baby after his 6 p.m. feed last night.

My breasts (not Rupert) woke me at 2.30 a.m. They were really engorged as a result of not feeding properly yesterday: I had expressed once, but should have done it twice, and Rupert's 6 p.m. feed had been shorter than usual due to his being so unsettled. I padded into the kitchen to get the breast pump. I was far too swollen to feed Rupert now (too difficult for him to latch on) and besides, he wasn't stirring yet, surprisingly. He's usually like clockwork during the night — waking 8 hours after the last feed, which would have made it 2 a.m.

After going into the nursery to check on his breathing (a common occurrence!) I went back to bed and expressed 100 ml. Still plenty left to feed him with but he wasn't awake! It was now 3.15 a.m. Don't want to wake him (even though on this occasion it would be more convenient) as we would like to train him to sleep through. Still, I worry about why he isn't stirring.

Went back to bed and read till 4 a.m. Still not awake! But he moved his head from side to side a few times. What to do?

Deciding that I might as well get some work done, I turn on the word processor, which is beside his cot. Will the noise wake him up? It doesn't (although he stirs), and I sit in the cold pre-dawn air, tapping away at my diary through yawns.

4.30 a.m. Still asleep. Ten and a half hours since the last feed — this has got to be a record! The poor baby obviously needs his sleep after such a wakeful afternoon. I think I'll have to go back to bed. If I do that, he'll wake for sure! I just hope he's all right.

5.00 a.m. Wake up with a start from a light but blissful doze, and dash into the nursery to put my face close to his. Still breathing. Still asleep! My breasts are hard and swollen again. Express some milk, and get to the 90 ml mark when I hear his plaintive cry. Awake at last! Eleven hours since the last feed! A well-rested baby, albeit an exhausted mother! Congratulations Rupert!

Sleeping through

Hopefully by the end of this month your baby will have started to 'sleep through'. Depending on whose figures you look at, roughly half of babies are sleeping through around the 3-month mark. What this really means is dropping a feed (or two) during the night. Baby may still wake briefly, but instead of crying he'll be able to put himself back to sleep, without disturbing you. What you're ideally aiming for is a final feed about 6 p.m., then a break of about 12 hours before the morning feed about 6 a.m.

Some parents may try to wake their baby for a 10 p.m. feed or top-up, in the hope that this will help them last through the night, but have trouble rousing the baby. This is because the early night sleep seems to be much deeper for a baby than day sleep, so it's better to try to get into the habit of giving the last feed, or a top up, just before it gets dark, say around 6 p.m. This should encourage the progression to the 12-hour break.

11 WEEKS

Rupert has started to notice and follow people with his eyes this week. When one of my friends came to visit, Rupert stared at her with interest for the first time and remained curious for the length of her stay. This morning Tristan was nursing him when I walked into the room talking, and Rupert turned to look at me — how flattering! And this afternoon when we took him to the local swimming pool (we wanted some exercise) he watched people walking through the entrance, turning his head to follow them as they passed. This kept him fascinated for ages!

He's smiling so much at his clown mobile (which hangs over the change table) that we've bought another musical mobile to attach to his cot, this time with furry animals (Tristan's favourites) instead of clowns. Although he shows no sign of tiring of the clowns, we feel a bit of variety is in order.

Last night he slept through again. That's three times in one week! (We hardly dare hope.)

Tristan and I both remarked today on how much easier it all is now. Today was a lovely relaxed day, a civilised start to the weekend. We had time to enjoy Rupert, and some time to ourselves. We feel in charge at last.

A father's view

Feeling left out

Fathers may be feeling pretty neglected by this stage. Little or no sex, no massages, cuddles, kisses or physical indulgences (or so it seems). In fact, you may be feeling like you are some sort of hired help. All because of that absolutely beautiful little bundle in the corner. Yes, you are being neglected — for a much better cause.

Baby's first mobile

Around this time your baby will be very interested in everything around him. Now is the time to increase the visual stimulation. Wind-up mobiles are great value. When you go shopping for a mobile, here are a few tips: have a look from underneath as this is the view your baby gets; choose one with bright faces or images; select one that clamps to the cot so it can be easily repositioned and keep the instructions. (They always look great in the shop but can be fiendishly difficult to put together.)

Handling baby

You can ease up on the 'extreme-care' handling procedures now, as your baby's neck muscles will be much stronger. However, babies are still pretty delicate and common sense should prevail.

Screaming phone calls

Imagine receiving an 'urgent' phone call while at work, lifting up the receiver and hearing only the unrelenting screaming of your child and the exhausted sobbing of your partner. At first I felt angry, annoyed that my wife could not cope and would selfishly burden me with her problems, when I had plenty of my own. And she was beyond even talking coherently to me about it!

Please don't make the same mistake. It was a classic cry for help from someone at the end of her tether. Catching my initial reaction I made what seemed like pathetic reassuring noises. 'Don't worry, it will all be better soon.' Basically I felt totally helpless. Should I dash home or call for help? If I got there would it all be over or ten times worse?

If you can, please dash home. If not, use those silly soothing words over again — they mean a hell of a lot.

Going out

If you are reasonably expert at coping with the baby, you're probably by now venturing out as a trio. If in a restaurant, you will be terribly self conscious about the baby crying. Resist the temptation to rush out the moment the baby cries. Instead, try some soothing techniques, or a bottle (the baby, not you). After all, you deserve a break by now, and there was no sign on the door saying 'No babies'. Commonsense should prevail. If it becomes a howling episode, grab some takeaway on the way home.

Much to your childless friends' amazement, you will be desperate to go home by 10.30 p.m. And you'll drink only a fraction of the wine. They will think you are behaving like some old couple. But then, they don't have to wake up at midnight, 3 a.m. and 6 a.m. (even on a Sunday).

Sleeping through the night

This is the big one. One day you will wake up, and instead of it being 3 a.m. and pitch black, it will be morning. Real morning, with light outside and the sounds of other humans going about their business. It's probably what Hillary felt as he crested the top of Everest. Just don't count any chickens. We had three amazing nights in a row, then went back to the old routine for the next month!

3 MONTHS OLD (12–16 WEEKS)

MILESTONES

- Reaches out and touches.
- Explores your face with his hands.
- Puts fists in mouth, plays with hands.
- Holds rattle when placed in hand.
- Lifts head higher and longer while on tummy.
- When pulled to sitting position, has little or no head lag.
- Focuses on things at a greater distance.
- Follows movement with his eyes.
- Vocalises (tunefully!) when you speak to him.
- May prop himself up on his elbows.
- May roll over from his back to tummy.
- May support own weight when held standing.
- Blows bubbles.

WHAT THEY NEVER TELL YOU THIS MONTH

- Baby shouldn't be offered solids for at least another month, as his stomach isn't mature enough.
- Drooling doesn't necessarily mean teeth are on the way.
- You can go back to work and continue to breastfeed.
- Expressing milk away from home can be difficult or frustrating.
- Postnatal depression can hit at any time.
- You may lose some hair from the scalp due to hormonal changes.

THINGS TO DO THIS MONTH

- Have a massage.
- Put your name down for a local day-care centre.
- Investigate insurance schemes to provide for your child's future school expenses. These are much cheaper if you start when he's a baby.

CHAPTER SEVEN

3 months old (12-16 weeks)

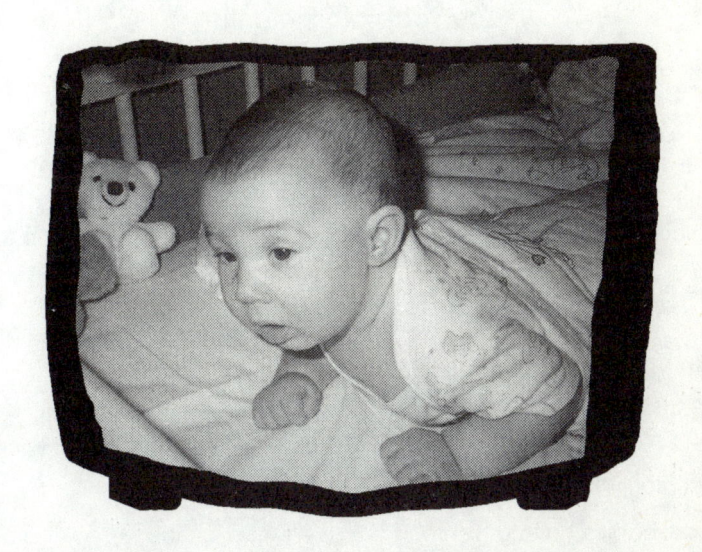

12 WEEKS

The magical 3-month mark and how things have changed. We have a real little boy on our hands now. We feel normal(ish). He's settled into a routine: his feeding times (5) are easily predicted, so are his restless periods. He sleeps like a log from about 7.30 p.m. till 5.30 a.m. or 6 a.m. (11 hours between feeds). Lucky us! Amazing how his body naturally adapts, and 'knows' to go without food breaks for the longer night-time sleep.

I must say, our being more organised and calm (in relation to the frantic confusion of the early days) certainly helps in dealing with the baby. Because now when he wakes up crying, instead of being flustered and anxious I simply hold him up in the air, look into his eyes, smile and say hello, knowing that (most times at least), he will stop mid-scream and smile back in delight. He just loves attention! Distracting him is certainly an art (I used to envy those mothercraft nurses who did it with such ease — now I can do it myself!).

Your baby this month

Now your baby is much more mobile, reaching out to touch, enjoying his hands, and really discovering his legs. When sitting with support, he has good head control. He can be happy for some time on his tummy, supporting himself on his arms and watching you. He may be babbling a lot, and starting to dribble. (If you're not yet using a bib, you may need to now.) He'll be awake for longer periods during the day. For the next couple of months he will probably average 12–16 hours sleep each 24 hours. His weight will probably increase by 150 to 250 grams each week, or $\frac{2}{3}$ to 1 kilogram by the end of this month. He's not yet ready for solids, although you can introduce them next month if you wish.

Some babies have developed a tousled mop of hair by now, but it's by no means 'the norm'. Your baby might have only a fine fuzz until he's about 12 months old.

12 WEEKS

Now that the dust has settled, the saying 'life will never be the same again', is really starting to hit home. I always seem to be running as fast as I can to try to catch up on everything I need to do. With daily activities built around Rupert's waking, feeding, caring and sleeping routines, there are no longer great chunks of uninterrupted time, just bits and pieces I grab when I can. More things to do, less time to do them in — what a catch-22!

I'm sure my friends must think I'm so rude for not contacting them more often, or arranging social gatherings, but there just never seems to be an opportunity. Sometimes I can envisage losing contact with the whole of humanity! Of course, that's why it's so different for the partner who goes off to work each day, unencumbered by the offspring. Busy, yes — maybe even frantic — but still able to enjoy those little taken-for-granted pauses and pleasures like a coffee break, a chat with an adult (without background crying), time to think and even the odd lunch!

Today a friend wickedly reminded us of our proud words uttered some time before the birth: 'The baby's not going to change our life — it's going to fit in with us.' We all laughed. No-one could have prepared us for this — or for the incredible joy he has given us.

Feeding and sleeping patterns

This is about the time when you may heave a big sigh of relief (like you might have done at 6 weeks), as baby seems to settle into a much more manageable and predictable routine. (Encourage this yourself by sticking to regular routines for baby as much as possible, for example, at bathtime and bedtime.) He may well be down to about 5 feeds a day, at intervals of between 3 and 5 hours.

Breastmilk or formula is all baby needs for nutrition until 6 months, although most people start solids between 4 and 6 months. Don't think about starting solids at 3 months, as baby's stomach is not yet mature enough, and he also runs a higher risk of developing allergies to certain foods.

By now, many babies will be sleeping through from the early evening feed until early morning (usually an 8–10 hour sleep). In addition, they will probably be having 2 or 3 sleeps a day, so they may sleep about 15 hours in 24. But remember, this is the ideal pattern, and it's normal for babies to have regular unsettled periods during which they don't sleep at all.

During the day, you may settle baby after a feed, only to find him waking, or stirring, again about 45 minutes later. Sometimes they can be like clockwork. This is because baby's natural sleep pattern, which has always been in cycles of 45–50 minutes, changes somewhat at about the 3-month mark. Whereas previously he slipped first into a light, dreaming sleep (the rapid eye-movement phase), now he goes first into the deep-sleep phase, which lasts about 45 minutes. When making the transition from this back to the dreaming phase, it's easy for baby to wake up. Hopefully by now you feel more confident about re-settling and helping baby put himself back to sleep.

12 WEEKS

When we came to check Rupert in his cot this morning, we found that he had reached out in his sleep and pulled over his teddy bear. How sweet they looked, cuddled together. And what a surprise, to find him capable of doing this.

So began a week of reaching for things, and actually exploring them with his new-found hands. He's discovered Tristan's face, and spends ages touching it, grasping at his glasses, and sometimes taking them off! While lying on the change table he reached for the clowns on his musical mobile for the first time, and we lowered it so he could touch them. He also spends ages with arms extended, examining his own fists with great interest, transfixed. And he even gets distracted from breastfeeding (only during the last half) by the colours of the cushions behind me, or the material of my shirt. He often grabs at my hair, and I have great trouble unclasping his little fingers. But it makes him seem so grown-up!

Cuddly comforts

Around this age, some babies adopt what is to become a regular source of comfort over the next few years. It's often a satin-bound blanket or cuddly toy. You may choose to anticipate this by providing baby with something suitable (convenient to travel with and not easily lost) or ignore it (my baby never became infatuated with one thing in particular). A 'cuddly comfort' may be a good substitution for a dummy or thumb.

12 WEEKS

How quickly 'good as gold' can change to 'absolute fiend'! Some days you see flashes of red, and feel like you'll scream if he doesn't give you some well-earned peace. You may snap at him, swear or perhaps pat him a trifle too heavily on the bottom while using your settling techniques. But minutes later, when all is blessedly quiet, you're mortified that you ever entertained anything but the sweetest thoughts towards him and you resolve to make it up as soon as he wakes, smothering him with apologetic kisses and soothing words.

Finally got Rupert to sleep just before Tristan arrived home (isn't it always the way?). Tristan bent over the cot to peer at the angel, and commented that it was still hard to believe he was all ours. 'Thank you, darling, for giving me the most precious gift', he said, putting his arm around me. And we both resolved, yet again, to never get upset or stressed when Rupert cried, but to remember how lucky we are to have him. Of course, it's easier said than done at times.

Play

Now that your baby's spending more time awake, you're probably wondering how to keep him entertained. This can be a challenge when baby has a short attention span, and is soon bored with one activity. Because he doesn't like to be alone for long, playtime can be labour-intensive. Instead of worrying about the work you could be doing, you might as well relax and enjoy it too!

Time on the floor is especially important now that baby is becoming more mobile. Allow him as much floor play as he'll tolerate, both on his back and his tummy, to help him develop skills for rolling, sitting and crawling. Give him toys in a variety of shapes and textures, so he can feel them and get different feedback from each.

Entertaining your 3-month-old

- Activity gym with a combined mat and play frame.
- Activity boards hung inside cradle or cot.
- Clothes airer with ribbons and toys dangling.
- Clear plastic balls with bells inside.
- Musical mobiles.
- Beans in a plastic bottle.
- Photographs covered in clear plastic, hanging from a frame.
- Onion bag with scrunchy cellophane inside.
- Bunch of bells from a craft shop.
- Mirrors.
- Safe kitchen items, like wooden spoons, plastic utensils.
- Wind-up swing, which baby sits in.
- Pram outside, or near the window, to watch fluttering leaves and trees.
- Portable chair, watching what mum is doing.
- Stand baby on your knee and bounce him up and down.
- Sit baby in a laundry basket, propped up against a cushion, with some of his toys.

13 WEEKS

Rupert's looking very cute and handsome, with thick glossy brown hair and permanently raised, perfectly chiselled dark eyebrows, framing enormous greeny-brown eyes.

We got out the photo album, and laughed at the shot of him leaving the hospital, a tiny vulnerable little thing curled up at the bottom of his baby capsule. Now he's bursting out of it! The many faces of Rupert — who would have believed there'd be so many different stages, in just the first 3 months?

He's developing at such a rapid rate with so many milestones still ahead. Each stage seems even more rewarding than the last, as his personality and accomplishments blossom. All my complaints about the crying, the posseting, the lack of sleep and time, the interrupted work, the frustrations pale in comparison to the joy and fulfilment of watching this radiant little being bloom, and of being part of a loving family.

Working and breastfeeding

Some mothers need to go back to work, at least part time, as early as 4 weeks; others may return at 3 months. And, of course, there are many who decide to take a break for a year or more. But if you do want to combine working with breastfeeding, there are a few points to keep in mind.

You *can* cut down your breastfeeds to twice a day — before and after work — if necessary. Some women are under the misapprehension that if you don't feed throughout the day you won't be able to maintain a good milk supply, but breasts are very adaptable. Some women can get away with not expressing any milk while at work (expressing can be difficult if you don't have the right facilities), but this usually means full, uncomfortable breasts, and the risk of mastitis (keep checking for hard lumps or red blotches). In any case, if you intend to feed your baby bottled breastmilk, rather than formula, while you're away, you will have to express in order to keep up the supply.

You *can* mix breast and bottle if necessary. For example, if you are working only 2 full days a week, you could choose to use formula for feeds while you're working, yet breastfeed normally on the other 5 days. This may not suit everyone, but it has worked for some mothers. Again, expressing while at work is recommended for breast health, although some women seem to get away without.

13 WEEKS

This weekend I had a freelance filming job so Tristan had charge of Rupert. His first stint as sole parent. Aha, I thought wickedly, this will be a chance for him to see first-hand what I have to cope with every day. And he thinks he's got a stressful occupation!

The job was about 20 minutes drive from home. My thoughts were often with my boys (father and son), and as often as I could I rang to see how they were. Tristan said Rupert slept like a log in the morning, and guzzled his bottle (expressed milk) when he woke.

I had already briefed my assistant on my need for at least half an hour's solitude in a convenient room about noon. At lunchtime I headed straight for an office far from the madding crowd, and brought out my 'expressing kit'. My breasts were very full and uncomfortable. I had to take off my suit (to avoid any risk of milk stains) and sit half-naked in the office, pumping with all my might. If they could see me now!

Sometimes the old expressing routine just doesn't go the way you want it to. Sometimes it takes forever to get the flow going, especially when you're under a lot of pressure, like I was today! Then it may only come out in a trickle, so that it takes ages to fill up a bottle (which of course you have to do, both to relieve your breasts and to collect enough to feed baby the next day).

I sat miserably in that office, pumping feverishly for a whole hour (oh, my aching muscles!), all for just 75 ml of milk, and the knowledge that my breasts would be uncomfortable again very soon. Everyone had finished lunch and was waiting for me, adding to my tension. I pride myself on being professional — how could I explain to them what I had been doing! I mean, if you'd mentioned expressing milk to me before I had Rupert, I wouldn't have known what you were talking about (sending it by courier?). To make matters worse, we were way behind schedule and there was talk of working on into the night.

My heart sank. This was just what I didn't need. It was bad enough working on the weekend, let alone when you need to breastfeed. I rang Tristan and asked him to bring the baby to the *studio at dinner time, so I could give him his last feed and get some relief at the same time.*

Tristan was spot on time, looking very pleased with himself for coping so admirably all day. I hugged Rupert, and was immediately aware of a familiar aroma. 'Where's his bag?' I asked Tristan. 'We'll have to change him first.' Tristan's face fell. 'Oh, I didn't bother to bring it', he said sheepishly. 'I thought we were only coming for a short time.'

Oh, the anguish! Here was the poor baby, jumpsuit wet with dribble, dampness starting to seep through at the other end, and a change of clothes and nappy nowhere to be found. And me desperate to begin a feed! A kindly co-worker (also a father) overhead our distress, and volunteered to dash out in search of an after-hours pharmacy, while Tristan looked after the baby and I continued to work. In 20 minutes (seemed like 2 hours) our saviour returned with nappies and wipes. We cleaned up the mess as best we could, but the baby had to stay in his damp jumpsuit while we fed. Poor Tristan resolved never again to leave home without the all-important bag!

Choosing a childcare centre

Unless you have a live-in relative or full-time nanny, going back to work means putting your baby into childcare. It can be a nerve-racking experience handing your baby over to strangers for a whole day or even half-day, so choosing a place you feel comfortable with is important.

I was lucky, in that the first childcare centre I found for my baby was a wonderful place, staffed by warm, caring people with the highest standards. They treated Rupert with loving concern and always took the time to give me a full report at the end of the day on his behaviour plus helpful tips on things I could be doing with him at home. They were happy for me to pop in during the day to breastfeed him. He was always serene and content, amused during his waking hours and patted to sleep at regular times in his own bassinet in a darkened room away from the noise and activity.

However, when I moved house and had to look for daycare in a new area I realised that not all centres were quite so perfect. I took Rupert away from one centre after just two weeks because I was not happy with the organisation of the place, the quality of care or the attitude of the staff towards both babies and parents.

So shop around until you find somewhere which satisfies you. After your initial visit, drop in unexpectedly a few times, in order to really gauge what the place is like, and make mental notes against your checklist. (See Childcare options, page 121.)

Childcare checklist

- Does it have a pleasant environment? A quiet street, lots of space, shady trees or verandas, outside play areas and good play equipment are all desirable but, of course, not essential. The essence of a good childcare centre is its staff.

- Is there a good staff–child ratio? There should be at least 1 staff member to every 5 babies.

- When you arrive, does someone come immediately to welcome you or are they all too preoccupied to notice?

- Do staff take time to answer your questions and discuss your concerns? At pick-up time do they communicate with the parents individually?

- Do the children look happy and well-occupied? Or are there lots of grizzly children and crying babies?

- Do the staff appear happy, pleasant and in control or are they frazzled? If staff seem hassled and lots of babies are crying, chances are the carers are not in control (or it's just a bad day!).

- Are the babies well cared for? Check there are no babies left to sleep unattended in hammocks or sitting unprotected in the sun. (Note that babies under 12 months should not have sunscreen applied.)

3 MONTHS OLD (12–16 WEEKS)

- What are the sleeping arrangements? Babies should always sleep in their own beds in a separate room away from the activity of the centre. There shouldn't be too many bassinets or cots crowded into one room.
- Are the older children well cared for? Are they wearing sunhats and sunscreen when they play outside?
- What's the catering like? Are the older children given natural, healthy food? Is it well-presented? Are they closely supervised during meal times?
- Are staff prepared to be flexible and responsive to your individual needs?
- When baby's on solids will the staff consult you before introducing him to new foods?
- Is the centre kept spotlessly clean? Check the kitchen and bathrooms.
- Is there a sensible structure to the day and is the daily routine posted up?
- How happy are other parents with the centre?

14 WEEKS

The days and weeks are slipping by so fast. This week Rupert has found his tongue — not to talk with, but to stick out! He spends much of his time grinning sheepishly, red tongue extended. And he's becoming so much more mobile! When he's lying on his back, he draws his knee up and presses his foot down, arching his back, in a valiant effort to turn himself onto his stomach. He's so strong that when he's in his portable chair he can push down with his legs and throw himself off balance.

Drooling

Around the 3-month mark, you may find your baby is drooling a lot and putting his fist in his mouth. He may continually have a soaked front, and develop a rash around his mouth and neck from the moisture. You'll probably wonder if there's a tooth on the way, but this doesn't usually happen until 4 to 6 months (although there have been rare cases of babies being born with one tooth!). It's probably just because his salivary glands are developing, and he's stimulating them constantly by putting things in his mouth. You may have to suffer the wet fronts for some time. Invest in lots of bibs, especially double terry towelling ones. This is when a baby pouch with detachable dribble bib (between your chest and baby's face) comes in handy.

15 WEEKS

> *This week Rupert's been grasping everything he can and putting it into his mouth — bibs, rattles, towels. He's now able to grasp and shake his rattles when we place them in his hand. When I gave Rupert tummy time in his cot this morning, he propped himself up on his elbows to say hello to the teddy bears at the side of his cot — a normal routine. But when he raised his head this time, I noticed he was holding it much higher and steadier than usual. (Has he been practising while I'm not looking?) Furthermore, he was gazing right over the cot bumper at the bright green filing cabinet beyond. What a development! Now he's aware of a world beyond his sleeping bay.*

Postnatal depression

Contrary to popular belief, postnatal depression is not something confined to the first weeks or months following the birth. It can happen any time up until your baby is two, although it often occurs between 3 and 6 months. You don't hear much about it, possibly because a lot of women don't even realise they're suffering from it, or they keep their feelings to themselves to avoid looking like failures. This just prolongs the misery.

Postnatal depression is entirely different from 'baby blues', which is a transitory condition common in the first 10 days, and passing in a day or so. Depression may last for a couple of months, or it may be a black hole that engulfs you for a year. It can break up marriages, and make you think you're going crazy. The most important thing is to be aware that there is such a condition, and that it can and should be treated.

Especially in the early months, when you're tired and edgy anyway, it's difficult to know what's 'normal' and what's not. Most of us are depressed at some stage, but if it's severe, you'll probably have a feeling that things are not 'right'. You may often be weepy, depressed, angry, frustrated, insecure, anxious, hopeless, confused, unable to cope, out of control; or even have suicidal thoughts or feelings of violence towards your baby. You may lose your appetite, be reluctant to go out, have sleeping problems or feel unable to adequately care for the baby.

Contact your doctor, child health nurse, family care centre or counsellor if you sense that you're out of your depth, and let them be the judge. Make sure it's someone who understands postnatal depression. Or at least call one of the telephone counselling services listed at the back of this book. It's not worth delaying to see if it goes away. Remember, too, that your tension can affect your baby and your partner, and create a cycle leading to more stress. Whatever treatment you're prescribed (it may be counselling, or a course of antidepressants), it also helps to have a support system such as family, friends, a mothers' group, or a family care centre. Get as much rest as you can, and arrange some time out by yourself. Make sure your partner understands the problem, and enlist his help.

16 WEEKS

He's almost turning over. When lying on his back, he levers himself up with his leg so that he's virtually on his side. And he can now turn himself around in his cot, so that his head faces the foot of the cot.

He's been gnawing furiously at his fist, and anything else he can find to put in his mouth, making frustrated noises (is he about to teeth?). He'll grasp toys from his gym with both hands to put to his mouth, and gets quite annoyed when he finds he's grabbed too many at once, or can't quite get a corner in his mouth!

Now that he's so mobile, it's becoming awfully hard to change nappies. I'll have to keep a supply of toys and other distractions on hand, to divert him from gymnastic practice on the change table.

A father's view

The baby bag

As the saying goes, 'Don't leave home without it.' Even if you are going out with baby for just 10 minutes, the bag is absolutely essential. Without a bottle, you cannot feed. Without a nappy, you cannot change. Without clothes, you cannot re-dress. Without the change mat, tissues, dummy, bib, safety pin, water, towel, rattle, booties, blanket, wet-ones, singlet or sun hat, you may be stuck with a very unhappy, crying baby.

If you are going solo, you may first have to win the confidence of your partner. Be prepared for a checklist that would not be out of place on the flight deck of a 747, along with constant checks and reminders. 'Of course, I remembered the nappies!' you will chide, as you desperately search them out. Be prepared. You will only forget this treasure-trove of practicality once.

School?

I was asked on more than one occasion which school our son would be attending, and had we booked him in yet. I assumed it was a joke. For some private schools, waiting for the birth would seem like waiting for the last moment. My advice? Everything in good time. (Of course, if you have an organised partner like mine, your baby will be on the waiting lists of 6 different schools before he's 6 months old!)

Playtime

Make sure you have plenty of time to play with your child and help him with his development, as he is now awake for much longer. Expect your baby to instantly discover a hitherto impossible action. One minute he is unable to reach out, the next he'll do it like an expert! It's yet another reason to always have a camera ready (your partner may not believe you otherwise).

4 MONTHS OLD (17–21 WEEKS)

MILESTONES

- May roll from back to tummy and back again.
- May push chest up and bottom up, but not together.
- May cut his first tooth.
- Grabs and grasps a dangling rattle.
- Real belly laughter.
- Vocalisation. He may make up to 4 different sounds such as aa, air, er, gl, kk, oo, ler.
- May double his birth weight.

WHAT THEY NEVER TELL YOU THIS MONTH

- Teething babies may bite your nipple while breastfeeding.
- Breastfeeding mothers may offer formula at some feeds without baby being adversely affected.
- If baby becomes unsettled, he may be indicating a need for solids.
- Don't leave baby in previously 'safe' places, like the change table or bed — his new mobility may take you by surprise.
- Don't invest in a baby 'walker'. These can cause injuries.

THINGS TO DO THIS MONTH

- Second round of immunisation.
- Visit your child health centre (18 weeks).
- Offer solids if you feel baby's ready.
- Start weaning baby off the dummy.
- Try baby water-awareness classes.

CHAPTER EIGHT

4 months old (17–21 weeks)

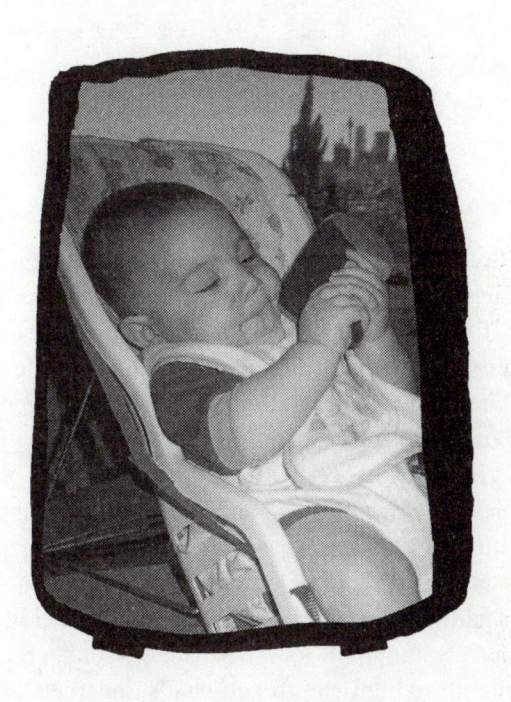

17 WEEKS

He did it! At last Rupert has managed to turn over — from lying on his back, to lying on his tummy. He had to strain to make it over the last bit! When sitting up on my knee or in his portable chair, he can now hold his head up unsupported for surprisingly long periods. He's also started to lean forward in his chair.

Your baby this month

This is the month of entertainment — a whole new era! He may lose a lot of his baby fat, and grow longer and leaner. He'll have a voracious appetite, and can now start experimenting with solids which heralds an easier time for you as far as breastfeeding or bottlefeeding and sleeping goes. Some babies will double their birth weight. Some will get a first tooth. Most importantly, at any time within the next few months, baby will work out how to roll over, and complete the feat before you know it.

Keeping your house in order

When well-meaning friends tell you to forget about the housework — that other things are more important, and your chores can wait — don't listen! If you let the house get really out of control, you'll find you're in over your head and you'll never catch up (unless, of course, you have a kind and willing mother, or can afford hired help). And that means even more stress.

The baby is first priority, certainly. But list your other priorities, and organise some time for these — perhaps while baby is sleeping, or playing by himself. Find your own balance, bearing in mind the mornings are always better for getting things done. You need to train yourself (and partner, if at all possible) to continually tidy items away, otherwise your dwelling will look permanently like a bomb site, and things will pile up so high you forget what's underneath them.

Hired help is not necessarily the answer, even if you can afford it. There are certain jobs that only you or your partner can do, like sorting through mail and paying bills. At 4 months, we were still discovering unpaid bills from the birth era, and important documents which should have been posted! Thank goodness we at least managed to keep the photo album up-to-date!

4 MONTHS OLD (17–21 WEEKS)

Entertaining a 4-month-old

- Rotate the toys as he'll get bored seeing the same ones continually.
- Check whether there's a toy library in your area. For a small fee you can borrow from a great range of playthings, which you can keep for a week or two, then swap for others to suit baby's changing needs.
- Buy a huge blow-up plastic beach ball. Place baby tummy down, over the ball, and roll him backwards and forwards. This will help develop his sense of balance and spatial awareness.
- Make your own toys with cardboard, string, streamers, scrunchy cellophane and empty plastic bottles.
- Show him kitchen utensils, saucepan lids and spoons.
- Read baby a simple book with colourful pictures and stiff board pages.
- From now on, baby takes special interest in his own reflection, so try putting him in front of a mirror.

Baby jumpers

The baby 'jumper' is a controversial piece of equipment. It's a cloth harness attached to an elastic cord (like a bungee cord) which hangs from a spring-loaded clamp on the door frame. The harness fits snugly around baby's waist and between his legs, suspending him with toes just touching the floor (so there's not too much pressure on the legs). In this position, baby is gently bounced up and down, and is free to push off with his toes and put himself into motion. On the first go, babies are quite surprised to suddenly find themselves upright and floating in space, but they seem to enjoy 5 minutes of gentle bouncing, especially to music with a good beat.

Many parents love them. (It provides a welcome diversion when you have run out of other ideas to amuse, and can give you a few minutes rest while baby practises his dance steps.) The manufacturers claim that jumpers develop skills, provide exercise, improve co-ordination and challenge curiosity. However, physiotherapists and child health nurses have serious concerns about their effect on development, and warn strongly against their overuse or misuse. They say baby is not ready to be in an upright position, as he has not attained his own balance in a still position; too much use can overstimulate baby's legs and feet, and lead to 'toe walking'; baby may jar his bones because he doesn't know how to land gently and bend his knees; it may affect the process of normal development; and if the equipment is not securely attached to the door frame, baby could fall and hurt himself.

Strong warnings indeed. Certainly, jumpers should never be used as a form of baby-sitting. Baby should always be closely supervised. You should not attempt this before baby's neck is strong enough to support his head — which may not be until 4 or 5 months, compared with the 3 months starting age recommended by one manufacturer. And baby should never be left on the jumper for more than 10 minutes at a time.

Baby walkers

These are a definite no-no. They don't help your baby walk and may even impede his development by depriving him of natural forms of movement. They give baby the wrong sort of mobility — allowing him to move around a room upright, supported within a frame on wheels and propelling himself by his toes, well before he is ready to cope with this sort of freedom. This can result in accidents both to items around the house and to baby himself. In the United States they have caused so many injuries to babies that they are banned outright; in Australia (at the time of writing), they just carry a warning.

17 WEEKS

Had to work today, and had booked Rupert into the creche but just couldn't seem to get out of the house! First he wanted a feed at the wrong time, then posseted repeatedly. I was kept busy changing sheets and clothes, while he cried and wanted to be entertained.

All this in between trying to make and answer necessary business calls, shower, eat and dress. At times, you just see red!

I guess there will be a big improvement when I'm no longer breastfeeding. What a release — I'll be able to put him in the creche and stay away for as many hours as I like, without the worry that he'll finish all my expressed milk and need the breast before I return! Oh, the blissful thought of no more pumping! And I'm sure sex will be a whole lot better when breasts are no longer associated with feeding.

Combining bottle and breast

Some breastfeeding mothers decide to substitute formula for one or more of the day-time feeds at this stage, in order to give themselves more freedom and flexibility. It means the baby can be left with grandparents or sitters during the day, without you having to worry about expressing milk or dashing home to breastfeed. (Mind you, pro-breastfeeding organisations would not approve of the practice.) For example, you may breastfeed early morning, give the bottle at mid-morning and then breastfeed in the afternoon. If you drop only one feed at first, allowing your breasts to adjust before dropping the next, then you may not need to express at all. (But always check for any lumps or redness, to avoid the risk of mastitis.)

Sometimes mothers who are intending to wean offer baby a little formula after the breastfeed, to get him used to bottlefeeding. This is probably frowned upon by the experts, but I'm told by mothers 'in the know' that it works beautifully, and their babies never reject the sneaky supplement. Many breastfeeding mothers wouldn't dream of offering anything but the breast, or at least breastmilk. Others give a formula substitute whenever it suits them, and manage fine. Do what works best for you and the baby — and feel confident about your decision.

Remember your child health centre

It's recommended that you pay a visit at least once between the ages of 4 and 6 months.

Apart from the professional advice and reassurance, it's good to meet up with mothers in the same boat as yourself, especially if you don't attend a mothers' group. Every other mother seems an 'expert' to whom you listen eagerly. It's amazing how much you can pick up from these casual chats.

If you intend to wean, consult your child health nurse for a program to suit you, in order to avoid problems with mastitis. She'll also advise on the best formula for your baby.

Problems with sleeping through

At this stage, your baby will probably be having between 12 and 16 hours sleep per day. This usually consists of the overnight sleep of 8 to 10 hours, plus 2 to 3 sleeps during the day, after feeding and play periods.

Many babies will by now be sleeping through from after the early evening feed to a decent time in the morning. But you may not be so lucky. I've known mothers who were still feeding at 2 a.m. or 3 a.m. at the 8-month stage. I have one friend whose son woke up every 3 hours for 2 years!

The point is, you can get help so why let it go on this way? If you've resisted seeking assistance so far, now could be the time. Sometimes the right book can be of benefit but, if not, see your child health nurse or family care centre, and get some first-hand advice on what's the best way to cope with your particular sleeping problem. It may be easy to solve.

Readiness for solids

Most parents are eager to try their baby on solids, although sometimes the 4-month mark sneaks up without you realising that baby is now old enough to at least have a go. If baby is ready, he may start to show an interest in what you're eating, or he may seem to be feeding constantly, or for longer, or be niggly after feeds. Perhaps he's not putting on enough weight. Sometimes babies who were sleeping through at 3 months (say from 7 p.m. to 5 a.m.) start waking again around 2 a.m. Most first-time mothers would not see a connection, but second-time mothers might well interpret this behaviour as a sign that baby is ready for solids. He may be. It's a matter of 'try and see'.

There's no need to try solids as early as 4 months, although it is advisable to introduce baby to them by about 6 months.

18 WEEKS

A cry in the middle of the night disturbed our sleep. The baby awake at 3 a.m.? Memories of the old days! This was surely a sign that solids were warranted from now on. Last week we tried him with half a teaspoon of cereal and expressed breastmilk, mixed to a paste. He wrinkled up his nose in mild disgust and gave an 'ugh' sound, but nevertheless swallowed it down. We had expected him to lap it up eagerly, so decided to wait until he showed a bit more enthusiasm.

This morning we brought out the rice cereal again, mixed with breastmilk — just half to one teaspoonful — after his morning and evening feed. He was a little surprised at the sensation, a little 'take it or leave it', but at least he didn't spit it out or react badly — the blob just sat on his tongue until it slid down of its own accord. He hasn't yet learnt the art of swallowing solids!

This evening, we caught Rupert sucking his thumb in his cot, like a real little boy. So now he knows how to find it (although he still seems to suck mainly his index finger or whole fist). Half an hour later, we discovered teeth! At least, some sharp little outcrops on the lower gums. No wonder he's waking in the night and irritable! And we thought it was hunger.

Starting on solids

This is an especially exciting period. One father told me that when his children started on solids they became, for him, 'real little people'. Starting on solids introduces a new era of freedom and convenience. Suddenly you find you can be more flexible with breastfeeds. If you're out, and baby's a bit hungry, it's so easy to top up with a few teaspoons of baby food or mashed banana. (Bananas are the most convenient portable food for babies and toddlers!) Sleeping and behavioural patterns may take a turn for the better. And now that breastmilk is no longer baby's only source of nutrition, breastfeeding mothers will feel happier about offering the odd bottle of formula if necessary.

Don't be in too much of a rush to give him food, though. Baby may not be quite ready, so test the waters gently, then wait a few days or more if it's not a success. You may even decide to wait another month before you experiment again, but don't delay too much longer — it's important to treat your baby to new tastes and textures.

My favourite starting foods were rice cereal and mashed banana — mixed with breastmilk (not cow's milk) or formula to a paste-like mixture. Rice cereal is a big favourite up until 6 months, because it's less likely to cause an allergic reaction than corn or wheat cereals, and it's iron fortified (baby's iron stores are now depleting). You could also try stewed apple, pear or avocado. Just see what takes baby's fancy. Some experts recommend starting off with strained vegetables (such as pumpkin, carrot or potato), rather than fruits, to avoid developing a sweet tooth (but it's debatable whether this actually works in the long run). Others advise not introducing vegetables until a month or so after starting on cereal, so you'll have to make your own choice.

Baby can either be on your lap or in a portable chair while you feed him. Put a little bit of food on a small plastic teaspoon, and deposit it well back on his tongue. He will probably be most surprised. Often more food will go out than stays in at first, so you'll have to have a bit of patience before you know whether it's a hit.

The golden rule is to go slowly. Offer only a teaspoon or two at first, and only one new food at a time. This way, you will know if baby has an allergic reaction to any of the foods. Many experts advise to always offer solids after a feed until about 6 months (so it doesn't interfere with his milk intake), while others say that once baby's established on solids it doesn't matter if he has them before or after, as long as he's a good feeder. I think the best time to start is after the morning feed. If that's successful, try it for a few days, then give him a little after the evening feed as well. Alternatively, stick to one meal a day and gradually increase the quantity, until you're up to a tablespoon or two. Then you could add a second meal.

At this introductory stage, quantity is not important, it's the experience that counts. By the time baby needs the food for nutritional purposes (at about 6 months), he will have graduated to a few tablespoons per feed, and a few feeds per day. You may reach this stage by the end of this month. And then he'll be on to new treats, such as sweet potato and peas.

When baby does take to his new regime, you'll possibly notice some other changes. Previously unsettled babies may become more settled; babies who were still waking for feeds during the night may now sleep through.

(See More on solids, page 218.)

Basic rules for solids

These are general guidelines, but keep in mind that different experts have different ideas about which foods to offer at various stages.

- Offer solids immediately after the morning and evening feeds.
- If baby is not interested, wait another week or two before trying again.
- Offer only a teaspoon per feed for the first few days then, if baby's willing, you can gradually increase to 2 tablespoons over the next few months.
- Most experts recommend you start with rice cereal, mixed with breastmilk, formula or boiled water.

- You might prefer mashed banana mixed with breastmilk or formula, or pureed cooked fruit such as apples or pears.
- Cooked vegetables, such as mashed sweet potato or pumpkin mixed with breastmilk or formula, can be next on the list.
- Start with one food only, then wait 3 days before trying each subsequent food, so you can check for allergic reactions (such as a rash around the mouth, irritability, unsettled behaviour, diarrhoea or wheezing).
- Never add salt or sugar to baby's food — his taste buds don't need it!
- While home-cooked, unadulterated food is best, buy commercial baby food jars for travel, picnics and emergencies.
- Save the tiny white plastic spoons that you get at takeaway places — they're ideal, because they're smaller and softer than ordinary teaspoons. You can also buy small spoons coated in plastic, specially designed for little mouths.

Teething

Teeth can appear any time after the first 3 months, earlier only in rare cases. Many babies get their first teeth between 4 and 6 months, although they can come as late as 12 months. You'll hear lots of horror stories about teething, but your baby may have no problems at all. You might notice lots of dribbling (although dribbling is common in babies and not necessarily related to teething). You may feel a bump on baby's gum. Or, like us, you may be taken by surprise with a sudden sharp nip on the breast or finger! (Some baby books will tell you that babies don't bite nipples. This is not true, as many of my friends can testify. One gave up breastfeeding abruptly when her baby started biting at 18–20 weeks!)

Baby will no doubt be putting everything he can into his mouth. Offer him a rusk or piece of crust (if he's on solids), or a plastic liquid-filled teething ring which is kept in the refrigerator. Generally, the use of teething gels with babies under 12 months is not recommended, because they contain aspirin which is not good for the kidneys (see a doctor first).

Some babies develop sore bottoms when teething. This is apparently because they dribble, and tend to swallow lots of mucus, which comes out as acid and irritates the skin. Plain zinc cream gives better protection than zinc and glycerine, as it stays on longer.

By the way, remember that baby's teeth and gums require cleaning. A clean, damp face washer or your finger is sufficient at the beginning. After a few weeks you can progress to a baby toothbrush with rubber bristles. Use water only for cleaning.

Possible teething signs

- constant dribbling
- dribble rash on chin and chest
- red swollen gums
- irritability
- biting
- flushed cheeks
- raised temperature
- sore red bottom, or rash
- loose, frequent stools
- poor appetite
- unsettled during night

19 WEEKS

Just one of those days ... Oh, the joys of motherhood! Didn't get to bed last night until about midnight, but then Rupert woke for a feed at 1.15 a.m. The next feed was at 6 a.m. Finally got him down, and managed to shower and eat before he woke for his next feed at 9 a.m. I had a busy day ahead. After feeding and amusing for two hours I put him down, only to have him wake again 40 minutes later. The day was slipping away, and I hadn't even started all the work I had to do!

I put him on the change table, but he was wriggling so much that he escaped his nappy and managed to cover himself in the mess. After cleaning up I placed the naked boy on the couch for a moment, while I spread a beach towel out on the floor to protect the carpet. But as I transferred him from the couch to the floor, I noticed he'd already left a soaking spot on the upholstery! Quickly depositing him on the towel, I raced for a cloth and returned to find him lying at the edge of a puddle of vomit. He grinned up at me in delight. ('I managed the hat-trick, mum!')

And so the day continues. Did I tear all that hair out, or did it just fall out naturally? When I finally got him to sleep again, after much grizzling on his part, it was only for half an hour — enough time to make a couple of phone calls and prepare (but not eat!) lunch. Six o'clock found me still trying to start editing my book, and I wondered what sarcastic answers I could give Tristan when he asked me his habitual question: 'How much work did you get done on the book today?'

The only time I get a free run is after 8 p.m. (that's when I'm usually preparing dinner), and by then there's not much time, energy or inspiration to devote to things creative and demanding. How do other people manage?

Oh, have I mentioned recently that Rupert's a gorgeous, delightful little boy and that when he smiles it's heaven?

Baby backpacks

If baby is becoming too big and heavy for the sling, and you do a lot of walking, consider a framed backpack. Now that his neck muscles have strengthened, he should really enjoy this form of transport. They're especially good for family outings, like bushwalking or a stroll around the park, when you don't want to have to cart a pram around. It's a good way for fathers to enjoy carrying their baby. Always remember baby's sunhat.

Miraculous mobility

It's around this time that your baby could catch you off guard with his new found mobility. You'll find him doing things you didn't realise he could do, like rolling from the centre of your large bed to the edge (and then falling off!), or wriggling off the change table. This can happen without any warning. Don't underestimate baby's growing gymnastic talents at this stage — and never leave him unattended in an unsafe place even for just a minute.

If baby does have a fall or a knock, it's wise to call your doctor to rule out concussion or other complications. Start investigating the availability of St John's Ambulance or other first-aid courses, for you and your partner, directed specifically at care of babies and children.

(See also Baby safety, pages 213–15 and Baby proofing, page 213.)

20 WEEKS

One of the delightful developments over the past couple of weeks is that Rupert can laugh. I mean really laugh, not just give a solitary chuckle, or a few giggles.

This afternoon I picked him up from day-care, fed him, and popped him into his cot for a few minutes while I finished a chore. I heard him grizzling, and bent over to give his foot a tickle. The distraction technique worked amazingly well — his sobbing turned immediately to laughter, which made me laugh, and then we just couldn't stop. We laughed at each other for a full 5 minutes!

I'm sure it's not a coincidence that he had spent today watching a group of toddlers playing and laughing. I think putting him into occasional day-care at this age is really valuable — otherwise he has to make do with just my company, and that has its limits!

Give your body a break

Soothe those aches in your shoulders or lower back, brought about by breastfeeding, expressing milk, carrying baby in a sling and lugging around the baby capsule. Book baby into an occasional care centre for a couple of hours, or call your mother in to baby-sit, and treat your back to an expert's hands.

- Find a good osteopath or chiropractor, making sure to check that they give a decent back massage as part of the treatment.
- Swedish or deep-tissue massage is a therapeutic alternative. Some masseurs will come to your house.
- Aromatherapy massage will treat your body and your senses, and transport you to another world. (Your partner may see it as a luxury, but we know better!)
- Enrol in a stretch class at a local gym (which may also have childcare).
- Try a water aerobics class, to lose weight and stress while limbering up.
- Ask your partner to baby-sit for half an hour before or after work each day, while you go for a brisk walk.

A father's view

Trying solids for the first time

It is probably about this time that *fathers* will experiment with solids. Why? Because you get to eat considerably more of every meal than they do! You will daintily show baby how an adult eats, and stare in disbelief as the little angel either wears it or drools it down his chin.

Everything he eats at this stage is bland. Everything tastes of nothing, and nothing tastes of anything. Stewed, mashed or congealed, it's all the same. This stage can be trying but all your patience and calm will eventually be rewarded with a smile and a gaping mouth. (A lot like those pictures of the young birds in the nest.)

The simple way to find out if he has teeth

He will bite you as hard as he can, then laugh at your reaction. I suspect that heavy dribbling is the anticipation of doing it again!

Social responsibility

If you drink socially, expect to sit on your wine for most of the evening. You will hardly drink when you go out and, if driving, you'll sit right on the speed limit and admonish those who drive exactly like you used to. Hindsight is a wonderful thing.

(Fathers') Attention Deficit Disorder

Your baby will probably spend most of his time with the mother, so he may give her all the best smiles, gurgles and intense loving looks, and ignore you. When you get home, your funny looks and sure-fire baby jokes may at best have your baby staring at the wall, ceiling or middle distance, but not at you. Don't despair, just persevere. You'll break through soon, and receive a priceless smile.

Making up for lost friends

'Do you have children?' is a question you previously would never have bothered to ask colleagues. But somehow there is a 'look' about a new parent (haggard, exhausted?), even if they are dressed in business attire, and are talking earnestly about important work issues. Just asking the question can make you some lifelong friends (to replace those singles you lost earlier), and your work-mates may be an enormous source of information if they have older children.

The witching hour

Work pressures don't always allow you to get home around dinner or bed time — often the most difficult time for mother and baby. Both are usually frustrated and exhausted by the end of the day. If you do get there in time, lend a hand and see the difference. Prepare dinner or bring home takeaway. Offer to bathe baby or look after him while your partner takes a bath. Iron a few of your own shirts if you don't already — and why not offer to iron for her as well!

You may have to take tissues to the movies

For many men this can be one of the most alarming consequences of fatherhood. For every film that features children, babies, separation and reuniting (and that means about 80 per cent of all movies), you will — when the parents, lovers, children, brother, uncle, dog, cat, mouse are finally united again — have to fight back tears. This, I am delighted to say, is only natural. Fortunately, most films have such a long list of credits that you have enough time to regain your composure. I now know why cinemas are kept so dark.

5 MONTHS OLD (22–25 WEEKS)

MILESTONES

- May pass toy from one hand to the other.
- Puts feet to mouth and plays with toes.
- Tries to push himself into sitting position.
- May raise chest and legs together by end of month.
- May rock on all fours by end of month.
- May maintain sitting position by end of month.
- May try to pull himself up to standing by end of month.
- May start on solids, if not already, or try finger food.

WHAT THEY NEVER TELL YOU THIS MONTH

- It's not too early to start reading to your baby.
- It's wise to continue with sterilisation of feeding gear after 6 months (although some books say not to bother) because bottles and teats are great breeding places for bacteria.
- A niggly or wakeful baby may mean he needs solids (or an increase in solids).
- Don't feed baby cow's milk, honey or egg whites until he's 12 months old.

THINGS TO DO THIS MONTH

- Start baby on solids (if you haven't already).
- If baby's on solids, expand the menu.
- Baby-proof the house.
- Do a first-aid course.
- Shop for a car seat, and have it fitted correctly.
- Shop for a highchair.
- Put baby's name down for a local preschool and private school if desired.
- If you're considering weaning, see a health professional for advice.

CHAPTER NINE

5 months old (22-25 weeks)

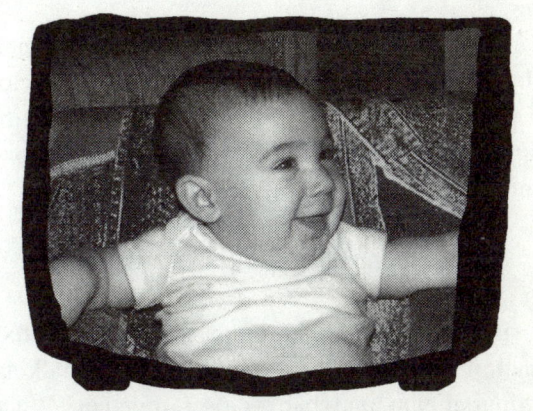

22 WEEKS

In days gone by we would put Rupert to sleep at the head of the cot, and find him in the same position when we checked up on him hours later. Not any more. He's started to favour turning over onto his back to sleep and sprawling diagonally across the middle of the cot. He's now a mobile little being! So independent!

Your baby this month

If you thought baby was mobile last month, wait until you experience the next few weeks. He is also much more aware. He may be able to sit and play contentedly with a toy for about 20 minutes. He will probably have doubled his birth weight by now. By the end of the month, his vision will be fully developed. He may reach the pre-crawl stage of rocking on all fours.

Introduce baby to books

Now is a great time to start reading to baby, although many parents wouldn't think of doing this at such an early age. I didn't, until a cluey aunt gave us our first stiff-covered nursery book. Get into the habit — why not encourage dad to read baby a story as his bedtime gesture? Baby may surprise you by actually paying attention, and looking at the pictures.

Browse around the children's section of the bookshop. Buy some of the simple, brightly coloured books with either cloth or thick cardboard pages — that way, baby can play with the book himself without ripping it to pieces. There are even plastic books which you can take into the bath.

Communicating with baby

Reading, singing and talking to baby are all direct forms of communication which help lay the foundations for talking later on, as well as bringing you and baby closer together. When you were pregnant you may have watched mothers in banks or supermarkets chatting away to babies who were obviously far too young to understand what they were talking about. Perhaps you thought they were mad. But by now you're probably aware that babies' minds are like sponges, absorbing things going on around them, even though they may not yet comprehend.

It's good to talk to baby while you do things, using a calm, clear voice. Repeat the names of items familiar to him, as well as those favourite words, 'mummy' and 'daddy'. Use games such as 'Round and round the garden, like a teddy bear', and rituals such as 'Bye bye'. You'll be amazed at how soon baby will start to understand and respond.

Baby proofing

Now is the time to plan ahead and start baby proofing your house, if you haven't already. Before you know it, your little baby will be crawling around the room, investigating every nook and cranny within reach (and some you didn't realise were within reach).

When planning your new kitchen arrangements, remember to allocate a cupboard or drawer for baby. Choose a low spot in which you can stack all your plastic containers, microwave dishes and other unbreakables, and also store baby's feeding dishes and cups here. He'll enjoy being able to rummage to his heart's content; and when he's a toddler, he'll appreciate being able to fetch his own cup and plate when he needs a snack.

Baby proofing tips

- Take all detergents, cleaners and other chemicals from under the sink and store them in a high cupboard, or invest in good childproof fasteners.
- Remove or secure sharp things and breakables.
- Store precious ornaments on high shelves.
- Buy a stairguard for use in doorways or with stairs.
- Buy a video guard, which clips over the front of the video, so that baby can't insert his fingers or toys.
- Get an electrician to install an earth leakage detector in your house if you haven't one already — this could save a life.
- Have all your power points replaced with safety power points, which prevent children sticking things in the holes, or buy push-in socket protectors for all points not in use. (See Baby shopping tips, pages 7–23.)

Safety tips

- Baby will now be reaching out to grasp things, with surprising strength. Make sure that any attachments to his cot, such as mobiles or hanging toys, are safe from his grasp, so there's no risk of choking or strangulation.
- Mosquito nets can be dangerous, as baby may pull it down and become tangled in it. Better to put flyscreens on the windows.
- Never leave baby sitting unattended in an upright portable chair, and never put his chair in a high place, like a table or benchtop — harnessed or not. You may be there with him, peeling the carrots, but in the few seconds it takes you to turn to the fridge, he could lean forward, tip the chair off balance and topple over, possibly falling to the floor.
- Never hold a cup of hot tea or coffee while carrying baby, and don't carry him too near to a stove or hot kettle. It's amazing how suddenly and strongly he can lunge from your hold.
- Never leave hot drinks near the edge of a benchtop or table. Baby may suddenly sneak up on you, and bring down the steaming cup all over himself. Often people dismiss these warnings as self-evident. Yet so often you see a baby in his parent's arms or in his pusher, within lunging range of a hot drink. And we keep reading of babies being rushed to hospital with disastrous burns caused by that 'harmless' cup of tea.
- Never leave a bucket full of NapiSan solution sitting on the floor, or within baby's reach. It is just too easy for carelessness or ignorance to result in a drowning.
- Buy a bath ring and a plastic bath mat to help keep baby safe in the bath. Obviously, never leave him unattended in a bath for a second, no matter how shallow the water. As well as the risk of drowning, there is now a risk he may attempt to pull himself up, and slip and fall, injuring himself in the process.

First aid

Both you and your partner should go along to a first-aid course. St John's Ambulance hold regular courses, usually a whole day or over several evenings. Your child health centre may be able to recommend a course in your area; and childcare centres are usually in touch as well. You'll never forgive yourself if an accident happens, and you didn't know how to best help your baby.

It's wise to brush up on these courses every year, especially through the toddler and preschool stages.

23 WEEKS

After absent-mindedly trying to turn down the volume of Rupert's crying (and realising, when nothing happened, that I was using the video remote control), I started to wonder whether I was going mad! Rupert seemed to have been howling non-stop all morning; not the usual crying, but screaming blue murder. It started straight after the breastfeed, when he should have been happy and content.

Recently he's been doing strenuous body exercises while at the breast (stretching my nipple in the process) and collapsing into misery on completion. Shows a terrible lack of gratitude. Maybe it's wind; maybe my breastmilk no longer agrees with him. But then, his crying always miraculously stops if I carry him to another room and give him a tour of the chiming mobiles, plants, or the like. Is he just a beastly little actor?

Anyway the crying, mixed with the inevitable posseting (no, that stage is not over, after all), nappy changing, struggles and frustrated efforts to prepare food and do a bit of work, took its toll. And, as usual, just when I'm reaching the end of my tether he'll stop, burst into sunny smiles and giggles, and my anger dissolves. Ain't nature wonderful!

I decided to give Rupert a bottle of formula, as an experiment, for the 2 p.m. feed. I'd never made one up before — I'd assumed it would be a bother, but it's so easy! Rupert didn't bat an eyelid

> *(I thought he'd complain and demand the breast!) but just guzzled it down contentedly. I was pleasantly surprised to find bottlefeeding rather a lovely experience, with its own special merits. Rupert felt cosy and placid in my arms. He didn't do his usual gymnastics. Afterwards, instead of grumbling, he sat and gooed while I burped him on my knee. Don't know what to make of it!*
>
> *It's hard to believe that he's almost 6 months. I'd always planned to wean at this stage, but now that we're here I'm a little reluctant, even though we'd like to conceive soon. The child health nurse said last week that it was good to breastfeed until the 9-month mark if possible. This gives baby the added protection of your antibodies until that time. Maybe I'll wean very gradually, and drop just one feed for the next month, to give me added flexibility. It means my breasts will adjust to supplying only 3 or 4 feeds a day, so I won't have to express while Rupert's in day-care.*
>
> *I just had a vision of Rupert as a tiny fragile newborn, nibbling like a mouse at my nipple. What a long time ago it all seems now!*

Adding formula to the diet

If you've stayed faithful to breastfeeding so far, now might be the time you're tempted to try an occasional dalliance with the bottle. After all, breastmilk is now no longer the only food to pass through baby's lips, so introducing formula no longer seems that great a sin — especially as you probably use it to mash baby's banana!

By now your breasts can probably cope with missing one feed without becoming uncomfortable. It means you can make up a bottle for the baby-sitter if you didn't have time to express, or let your partner take over feeding duties occasionally as a special treat (for everyone). I'm not suggesting you make this a habit — it's just good to know you have the flexibility. If you're planning to go back to work soon, you should start getting baby used to the bottle anyway, whether it's with formula or expressed milk. Some mothers will choose this time to start weaning (in other words, take baby off breastmilk altogether). Remember to seek some professional advice beforehand (see When to wean, pages 224–5.)

24 WEEKS

By late morning the day had turned frantic. Rupert vomited on his quilt and started crying. I mopped up, then harnessed him into the Jolly Jumper. Just as I bent to place a protective towel under his feet he vomited again, all over the carpet. He started screaming. Silly me for putting him on the Jumper when he'd been posseting. I mopped up again and struggled to untangle him from the Jumper while he wriggled the other way. I tried to make some toast for brunch and get ready to go out. Rupert kept crying. I changed his nappy, undressed him, and forced on a new jumpsuit. He posseted all over it. The screaming became deafening as he fought to eject himself from the change table. Tears spurted from his eyes. Tears of frustration began to spurt from mine. I pleaded with him to be quiet. I shouted at him to shut up. It was all reaching breaking point.

Mercifully, Tristan dropped in at that instant for a lunch break and took over while I tearfully got ready to run my errand. The skies clouded over in empathy and when I returned an hour later, refreshed by the break, it was pouring rain. Then Tristan left for work.

Rather than spend the rest of the afternoon trying to entertain a grumpy baby, I decided to visit Susanne, whom I'd met in prenatal classes, and her baby Bonnie. Bonnie's a pretty little elfin creature with wispy blonde hair. Rupert, of course, towers over her, despite being 2 weeks younger. She fixed me with a dazzling smile, while Rupert grinned cheekily up at Susanne. Then Rupert reached out and grabbed Bonnie's ear, before trying to wrench off her polka-dot jumpsuit by the neck. Bonnie regarded him with wary fascination. We put them on the floor to study each other and their toys, while we launched into a discussion on baby foods, sleeping patterns and regaining our figures! Two active professional women, both in the same industry, and we didn't once touch on the subject of work! Who would have thought it possible!

Test baby's hearing

Even if you've been having regular checkups at your child health centre, it doesn't hurt to do your own test. Make a sudden loud noise, or call out, and see if he responds. He should turn his head — if not, consider a checkup.

More on solids

Until now, baby hasn't needed solids for nutritional purposes, although it's been a good opportunity to experiment with tastes and textures. Over the next few weeks you may notice that milk alone isn't satisfying your baby like it used to, or that he needs more than before. He may become niggly during or after feeds, or wake up during the night. He may open his mouth or move his tongue when watching you eat. Be aware of the signs that you should be either beginning, or increasing, his intake of solids. If he's crying inexplicably straight after a feed, try offering a teaspoonful of something. You'll soon know if hunger is the cause.

Nutritionally, it's best to start on solids within the next month or so, if you haven't already.

There are some mothers who, consciously or not, delay the introduction of solids for as long as possible, either because they like being the sole supplier to their child, or because it signifies their little baby is growing up. Others, who started off at 4 months, religiously obeying all the instructions (a teaspoonful after the morning feed), forget that baby's intake of solids needs to be gradually increased over the next few months.

Expanding the menu

If you're just starting baby on solids, see pages 200–2 for the basic guidelines. If baby's now into his second month, it may be time to introduce cooked vegetables if you haven't already. Mash potatoes and pumpkin, and blend other vegetables such as peas and carrots. By now baby may be taking up to two tablespoons per feed. Remember to offer each new food individually at first, and wait a few days before you add the next to the menu. Start easing baby into the 3 meals a day routine, by offering solids at lunch-time as well.

You'll find that the experts differ widely in their advice about what foods to give and when to give them. Some professionals advise not to offer foods other than cereals, fruit and vegetables until baby's *at least* 6 months. Others say it's now okay to try foods such as full-fat natural yoghurt, grated cheese, or a little mince meat, poached fish or chicken blended in with the vegetables. So you'll just have to follow your own instincts, or see what works for other mothers.

The contradictory advice continues with finger food. Some experts say not to give finger food until about 8 months. Others tell us that babies who refuse food unless they can feed themselves, can be introduced to finger food as early as 5 to 6 months. This includes grated apple, small bits of paw paw, fingers of toast and steamed vegetable sticks. From my observation, second babies tend to enjoy such delicacies at an earlier age than first babies — older siblings set an example, and seasoned mothers tend to be more adventurous and flexible with the rules.

One thing everyone seems to agree on is that egg whites (possibly causing allergies) and honey (possibly causing infections) are out until baby reaches 12 months, along with cow's milk. All types of nuts, and crunchy peanut butter, are off-limits until your child is 5 years old.

Freezing solids

Mash or puree a large quantity, freeze in ice-cube trays, then transfer cubes to a freezer bag — or store in small plastic containers with lids.

Some foods, such as potato, need to be mixed with another vegetable to freeze properly.

Label with the date, and use within 2 or 3 months.

Feeding bibs

Now's the time to buy one of those hard plastic bibs, with the curved lip, or trough, for catching all the drips and missed pieces of food. They're not attractive (especially when you see them in action!) but come in handy at home. You simply rinse them under the tap and re-use.

25 WEEKS

My morning at Tresillian's day stay clinic was invaluable as usual. I sat down in the playroom and talked with the nurse while Rupert examined some toys, his mind taken off the 10 a.m. feed now due.

'Why does he cry in between and immediately after breastfeeds?' I asked.

'He wants solids', said Kate promptly. 'Milk alone is no longer enough to satisfy him and he's probably a bit bored with it by halfway through the feed.'

How obvious! I'd been waiting up to half an hour after the feed to give him his solids, but his stomach was demanding them immediately.

'That's also the reason he's waking up so early in the morning', added Kate. 'He should sleep until at least 6 a.m.'

'Thank goodness,' I said. 'These 4.30 a.m. starts are tiring us out, especially as Tristan and I can never seem to get to sleep before midnight. We don't start preparing dinner until after Rupert goes to sleep. This is usually about 9 p.m., so we find ourselves eating around 10 p.m., sometimes later.'

'That's not on,' said Kate, much to my relief. 'He should be going to bed about 7 p.m.'

What a wonderful vision. Baby fed and bathed at 6 p.m., read a story (yes, even at this young age), and then retiring to bed, leaving the evening free for his tired parents to do what they will! Apparently I haven't been feeding him enough — quantity or variety. Still following the directions for 4-month-olds, I've been giving him a couple of tablespoons of pureed fruit or vegetable 3 times a day. But as he's virtually a 6-month-old now, he should be having a decent bowl full, with lumps, rather than a smooth puree. This must be a fairly common oversight. One of the other women there today had a 9-month-old boy who was being fed the same as Rupert — mostly breastmilk, but the occasional pureed solid, in small quantities. She admitted sheepishly that she was still thinking of him as a 4-month-old baby. And this woman had a 2-year-old as well, so experience obviously doesn't mean automatic know-how!

Kate suggested I try giving Rupert solids first, to avoid the whingeing at the breast syndrome. So this afternoon I mixed the rice cereal according to her directions (twice as much as usual) and he scoffed down the lot, then transferred to the breast. No crying. Score one point to Kate.

But so much for going to bed early! It seems impossible for Rupert to actually go to sleep before 9 p.m. Both last night and tonight we tried putting him in his cot around 7.30 p.m., as Kate suggested, but he was full of beans and alternatively played and grizzled for the next hour. I guess we'll keep on trying.

Shopping for a highchair

Like me, you may have associated this piece of equipment with much older babies, not realising that your baby may be ready to graduate! Depending on baby's sitting abilities, you may choose to move baby to a highchair any time between now and 9 months. When you're dealing with solids, it certainly makes life easier. Remember to also buy one of the special foam supports, to help keep baby upright.

Shop around to see what's on the market. You may find versatile pieces like a combination highchair, rocker and play chair, brightly coloured, and complete with steering wheel at ground level for baby to play with when he's on the floor. Another good buy is the combination high and low-chair: comprising a standard highchair which either comes apart or converts to produce a low-chair with wide table — it's great for sampling solids from a safe, stable position, and for playing with toys while upright.

Important points to look for in a highchair are stability, a secure, well-fitting safety harness, and a large tray which is easy to place over baby's head, and easy to clean. Look for a tray which curves up at the edges, with no corners or crevices to harbour crumbs and germs.

A handy item you may like to invest in later is the legless chair, which clamps onto the tabletop. It's demountable, and especially useful for restaurants and travelling. It really makes a difference if baby can sit up with the family, rather than being relegated to a stroller, or held wriggling on your knee.

25 WEEKS

Today I bought a highchair for Rupert. What bliss to be able to secure him while I prepare his meal, and hear him playing happily with his toys on the new tabletop. And then the luxury of feeding an upright strapped-in baby, with a surface on which to place his dish, instead of the wriggling little eel who used to get mashed food all over him and us!

The desperate decision to buy the chair came this morning, as I was reheating the same cup of coffee in the microwave for the fourth time. I could wait no longer. There are times when I can't leave him to just roll about in his cot or on the floor, particularly after a breastfeed when he's likely to posset if left horizontal. Today I spent from 5.30 a.m. till 3.30 p.m. on virtually continuous baby soothing duty — he slept for only about an hour during that time!

It was a hideous day. It started off on the wrong foot when Tristan had to do some computer print-outs in the office/nursery at 7 a.m. (just after I had put the baby down), and Rupert's normal sleep pattern was disturbed. I had planned to have a nap, but ended up helping Tristan with his work instead. He sailed out the door at 8 a.m., leaving me holding a very niggly baby. It was one of those mornings (rare, thankfully) when I tried everything in turn, but nothing seemed to work. Was he hungry? Tired? Bored? Teething? Feeding times went awry, and so did my schedule. I found myself resenting Tristan's escape, and angry that it always seemed to be my work that went by the board. When 2 p.m. came and he was still awake (though zombie-like), I bundled him into the car and down to my local baby shop.

Sandra, the proprietor, had put aside a chair she highly recommended and, after looking around myself, I agreed with her choice. It's a highchair which doubles as a low-chair and table. There are several different types on the market, but this one stands out. It's very easy to manage, with the highchair simply lifting off its base to become a low-chair. The base then upends into a separate table, which will be invaluable when he's a little older and into scribbling and other activities.

At present, all we really need to use is the low-chair, which has an extra-wide tray. This means I can sit on the floor or an armchair to feed Rupert. When he's alone in the chair, I don't have to worry about him falling from a great height. Not that he's likely to fall — this chair is extremely stable with sturdy legs, and has the added advantage of straps which fit snugly around his waist and attach to the crotch strap. With some models you have to buy a separate harness while others have the straps too low, so they fit around his hips and don't provide enough security.

So, the new system is bliss. Much as I liked the look of the wooden chairs, the practicality of this chrome and vinyl model outweighs all other considerations!

When to wean

There's often some confusion between the term 'weaning' and the introduction of solids. Weaning means taking baby off breastmilk and accustoming him to either formula or replacement food. You can combine breastmilk and solids for many months, which does not necessarily mean the baby is being weaned.

Breastfeeding mothers who are trying to get pregnant again often decide to start the weaning process at 5 or 6 months, to give themselves a better chance of conception. (Contrary to popular belief, breastfeeding is not a foolproof method of contraception.) It's a convenient time to wean, because it coincides with the solids phase. A combination of solids and formula also means much more freedom and flexibility for you.

Although breastfeeding to 6 months means you've given baby good protection against infection and allergies during his most vulnerable period, most breastfeeding advocates recommend continuing to 12 months if you can, at which time you can change to cow's milk. If you make it at least to the 9-month mark, you have the added advantage of being able to avoid bottles altogether, progressing straight to a training cup. It depends a lot on whether you're enjoying the experience. Some women quite happily breastfeed until their children are toddlers, and even then are reluctant to give it up.

How to wean

You may feel you don't need any help, yet child health nurses strongly advise that you consult them before starting, to set up an individual program depending on your needs, and avoid problems such as mastitis. They'll also advise on a suitable formula. The Nursing Mothers' Association will also give you advice.

If you want to start now, allow about a month for the whole process. That's following the routine of skipping one breastfeed, say the lunchtime one, for one week, replacing it with a bottle then dropping a second feed the second week, and so on. It's practical to leave the early morning breastfeed till last, as that's when you have most milk,

5 MONTHS OLD (22-25 WEEKS)

although you might prefer to keep the evening feed, if it helps you settle baby at night.

Drugs are no longer prescribed for weaning, as your breasts will adapt to the new routine if done gradually. (Gradual weaning is best for your breasts and less traumatic for the baby.) Express a little milk at feed times if you're full or uncomfortable, and massage breasts under the shower. Be aware of the signs of mastitis, just in case (see pages 79–80).

For babies under 9 months, going from breast to bottle is probably a smoother and more comforting transition than going from breast to a training cup. Some babies over 6 months, however, may be able to skip the bottle altogether, if that's what you prefer to do.

A note for those who plan to keep on breastfeeding. What they never tell you, laments one of my friends, is how to wean a 2-year-old who steadfastly refuses to give up the breast — and is too smart to believe that your breasts have 'run out of milk'. You'll understand the problem if you've ever witnessed a burly demanding toddler ripping off mum's dress in public, and refusing to take no for an answer! You'll need to find a book on toddlers if you want to know how to solve this one!

Weaning off the dummy

Some babies will cease using their dummies of their own accord; others will continue till they're at preschool if you let them. The solids phase could be a good time for you to start easing up on dummy use, if it's well established. Give him a rusk to suck instead!

From capsule to car seat

Moving from baby capsule to car seat is a landmark indeed, a delight for both you and the baby. Although the official changeover time is 6 months, parents of large babies often find the capsule too much of a squeeze long before then. Babies can use a car seat if they weigh

9 kilograms or more, measure 70 cm in length or can hold their head erect — or at six months, whichever comes first.

Instead of being crammed in and helpless on his back, baby will now be able to look out of the window at the passing traffic and feel part of it all. And still nod off to sleep when appropriate. Make sure the seat's adjustable, so it can be tilted back at first for baby's comfort. You may also like to buy a foam or inflatable neck support to stop his head flopping to the side during nap time.

Toddler Kindy Gymbaroo

There are a few different organisations which offer gymnastic activities for babies — theoretically from 6 weeks of age, although most prefer waiting until at least the pre-crawling stage. Toddler Kindy Gymbaroo is probably the most well-known baby and toddler gym, established in 1982, and now with centres throughout Australia. Its aim is to 'enhance the learning abilities, behaviour and health' of the children, helping them to achieve their full potential. The classes are based on scientific studies which show that early movement stimulation aids in maturing the nervous system. They say that many problems later in life, even illiteracy, may be caused by a lack of motor development skills and co-ordination in infancy; in other words, not enough 'sensori-motor' experiences like crawling, creeping, balancing, rocking, spinning, hanging, rolling and the like.

Staff frown upon practices or equipment which can interfere with normal development, like bouncinettes, walkers and excessive use of playpens. The good thing is that the centres also act as watchdogs, observing the children, and looking to prevent later school learning problems.

Classes are held every week, usually in a community hall with gym equipment, and last for half an hour. After some group activities, including singing and movement, you help your baby participate in selected activities centred around different skills. As well as improving baby's physical (and apparently mental) prowess, it can be a fun outing for you both, and an opportunity to meet other new parents and playmates.

25 WEEKS

This afternoon Rupert went to his first session of Toddler Kindy Gymbaroo, held at a local church hall set up like a gymnasium. He's in the 'pre-crawling' class, supervised by Joanne. There were eight mothers with their babies, most aged 6 or 7 months. Rupert stared around him in fascination, mouth open. I've decided he's the observant, rather than the demonstrative, type (takes after his father).

It was surprising how different the babies' rates of progress were. Some had teeth, some were sitting, and some were already crawling (although 'crawlers' are theoretically the next class up). Joanne stressed that at this stage there are no set standards, so you shouldn't worry about your child being 'slow' or 'fast' to develop.

We started off sitting on mats, valiantly attempting different massage techniques on our wriggly babies (all excited at the presence of other noisy little creatures like themselves) and maintain eye contact. Then we did some (well-supported) somersaults, which help develop the baby's sense of balance, followed by nursery rhymes with actions. Was this really me, trying to remember the words of 'Twinkle Twinkle' and 'Hickory Dickory Dock'? To me it seemed pretty early to start them on songs, but apparently something rubs off. And Joanne says that if you play 'peek-a-boo' games with them using a hanky or scarf, they'll soon learn to pull down the cloth themselves at the appropriate time.

Joanne put on some music so we could all have a jolly dance, swinging the babies around as much as possible. Rupert just adored this — his eyes shone and his little face was one great smile. What a revelation.

The next stage was free play on the kindy equipment with each mother holding her baby as he rolled down a padded vinyl incline, rolled on a vinyl log or large ball, rocked on a hammock, bounced on a trampoline or hitched a ride tummy down on a skateboard. Rupert took delight in them all.

> We finished the 40-minute session with some more songs, waving a large, brightly coloured parachute for visual stimulation. I can see this is going to be a valuable means of keeping me informed of ways to help the baby's development, as well as the obvious benefits for Rupert himself.

Entertaining your 5-month-old

By this time, you may be running short of ideas to entertain baby. When his positions are limited to rolling about on the floor or sitting restrained in a chair or pusher, you start feeling a bit constrained, especially if you haven't got 'live' entertainment, like older siblings playing in the same room. Try some of these activites:

- Play peek-a-boo.
- Sing nursery rhymes.
- Read stories.
- Dance with baby to lively music.
- Bounce him gently on your knee.
- Roll him on a soft mat, one way then the other.
- Videotape baby or record his voice, then play it back.
- Sit him in high or low-chair with toys or mobiles.
- Buy him some baby musical instruments.
- Lie him on his tummy in front of a mirror, with toys.
- Sit him in front of a window, or outside, to watch birds, cats, trees, the movements of light and shade.
- Take him to the playground to have a slide or swing on your knee.
- Take baby to a coffee shop, and have a break too.

Playgroups

Usually you're either a 'playgroup person', or you're not! It depends a lot on how social you are, whether you already have a support group, and whether your child has his own peer group companions in the form of friends, neighbours or relatives. Also, of course, not every mother will have the time to while away a morning a week chatting with other mums or be able to commit to morning tea or play duty on allocated days.

At this age, playgroups are probably more for your benefit than baby's, offering you warm, supportive company, a few hours of hassle-free relaxation, the chance to share like experiences and problems, and the opportunity to establish yourself in a group where baby will be able to grow older with playmates, while you make long-term friends.

Water-awareness classes

Some people call it 'baby swimming' class, but we certainly didn't get to that stage. If you have the time, and if there are sessions nearby, then it can be fun to get baby used to the water. Specialist baby and child swimming centres may take babies from 3 months, although 6 months is recommended as the ideal starting time. Before this they can just as easily practise in the bathtub at home!

At 5 or 6 months, baby has no fear of the water: he is becoming more social; he hasn't reached the 'separation anxiety' stage, so he is comfortable with teacher contact; and he can be taught to float independently on his back. Sessions are held in small groups, in a warm pool about a metre deep, with baby and parent participating together. Mind you, it's a bit hard trying to teach them things when they don't understand or respond to instructions! And even if you do get them to the swimming stage, many babies go through a 'fear of water' phase some months later, only to regain a love of water when they're toddlers. So if you decide to wait and start them when they're one or two, you probably won't have missed out.

School and preschool

When your baby is less than 6 months old, preschool seems a long way off. But it's wise to think ahead, because some preschools have long waiting lists. Even if you're unsure where you will be living in a few years' time, it doesn't hurt to make provisional arrangements. Investigate the kindergartens or preschools in your area, and find out their requirements.

If you're going back to work soon (or already working), you might have enrolled in a childcare centre. Maybe this is a centre which caters for children over 2, as well as babies, which means your child could stay on until he reaches school age.

If you plan to stay at home with your baby, looking at childcare centres may seem unnecessary. However, when baby is 2 or 3 you'll probably want to enrol him in a kindergarten or preschool — the terminology changes from state to state — even if just for half a day per week. The company of other children and adult carers will provide him with valuable socialisation skills, while the stimulation and daily schedule will help equip him for school life. And, of course, it gives you a much-needed break.

Depending on where you live, you may have a local kindergarten which takes children on certain days according to their age; or a kindy or preschool which operates like a long day-care centre, taking children from 2 to 5 years, 5 days a week, often with a minimum requirement of 2 days per week. There are also alternative learning centres, such as Montessori, which keep shorter hours.

At around 5 years of age, your child will start school. Confusingly, this first year (before first grade, or year one) may be called preps, preschool or kindergarten, depending on which state you live in.

If you are contemplating sending your child to a private school or, indeed, to any school with a waiting list, you need to put your name down now. Beware, you may have to make a hefty deposit. Some private schools have large deposits to deter parents from applying to numerous schools, and only making their decision at the last minute, thus falsely inflating projected school enrolment figures.

5 MONTHS OLD (22–25 WEEKS)

It might seem ridiculous to think about school when you are looking at a tiny baby. Schools can vary considerably in quality over a decade, and so can your income. However, it's worth doing a bit of quick investigation at this stage. Buy a book on local schools, talk to your child health nurse and parents of local school-age children, and discuss the issue with your partner.

A father's view

Congratulations! You've done it! You've survived 6 whole months, and your little baby will soon transform into a *toddler*! A whole new world of challenges and delights awaits! But the initiation period is over, and most parents now blithely toss away their baby books, preferring to go by intuition or what other parents say, until they're again in urgent need of reference material for the Terrible Twos!

Take time off for those milestone paediatric checkups
For fathers, going along to the regular checkups at the child health centre or paediatrician can be immensely valuable. It's an opportunity to check that your child is really miles ahead of all the others, that he is a genius, and future world champion in everything. It's really good to be able to ask questions about current development and general health, and assess what is going to happen in these areas in the next 6 months.

Safety tips for fathers
By now your baby will be surprisingly active — one minute sweet and placid, the next squirming to escape or grasp an object. If you are baby-sitting, don't leave him unattended or on a bed, change table or benchtop (even in a portable chair or bouncer), as this is the age when babies can easily topple. Check the area around the cot, too. With such a surprisingly strong grip they can pull things down on themselves. (Parents with long hair hardly need reminding about the tenacity of a 5-month-old's grip.) Their speed will also surprise you!

A word on changing nappies from now on
Your little angel will (if he hasn't already) turn into a wriggling monkey, intent on grabbing and experimenting with everything, and I mean everything: lotions, liquids, ties, best shirts, and the contents of the nappy are all literally up for grabs. His willpower is developing at an equally alarming rate. You will need about three and a half hands

to subdue and conquer during nappy changes. Your last resort may be calling attention to the change-table mobile, if it hasn't been pulled down already. You can adopt the 'Blitzkrieg' method and stun him into submission with your speed and sense of absolute purpose. Remember, you are allowed to say 'no'.

Read stories

Reading stories is great fun and a great habit to get into for everyone concerned. If you've never ventured into the children's section of the library or book store, do it now. Even though your child cannot read or understand what you are saying (just as well sometimes), he'll love the interaction and attention, and may hang on every word you say — perhaps it works on some deeper level.

Some babies have amazingly short attention spans and will be staring around the room after page one. But persist — you're setting patterns for future years. Start with something short and simple, preferably with cardboard pages, so those little hands can 'help' without ripping the pages (that comes later).

Sing a lullaby

If you can play an instrument or sing both you and the baby are fortunate. Even if you're not musical, treat baby to a song. Babies are surprisingly non-judgmental. They just love *you*.

6 MONTHS AND BEYOND

MILESTONES

- Reaches out his arms for you.
- Holds his own bottle.
- Can start drinking from training cup.
- Maintains sitting position.
- May start to crawl.
- May pull up to standing position.
- May cruise around room holding on to furniture.
- Responds to his name.
- May say first words ('dada', 'mama', or even 'more'!).
- May get some teeth (if he hasn't already).
- Can fully focus eyes and has peripheral vision.

THINGS TO REMEMBER

- 6 months: third immunisation
- 9 months: child health centre checkup
- 12 months: immunisation for measles, mumps, rubella

CHAPTER TEN

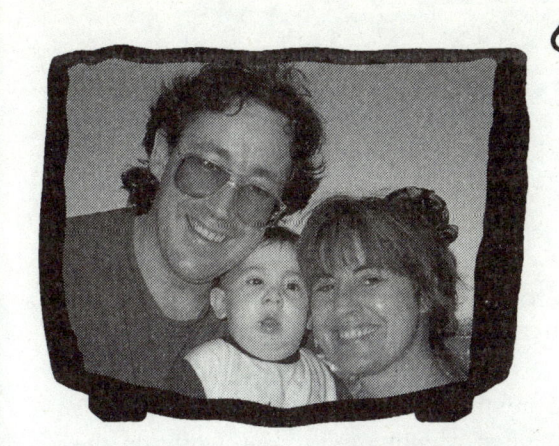

6 months and beyond

7½ MONTHS

Tristan came rushing into the kitchen to chastise me, as I was making Rupert's bottle.

'Darling, you shouldn't leave him alone like that!'

'Like what?' I asked in dismay, following Tristan into the livingroom. There stood Rupert, balancing upright in wobbly fashion against the couch, head turned towards us, grinning happily.

'But I left him on the floor ...' I started, then wondered if Tristan was up to one of his tricks.

We looked at each other and realised we were both just as surprised. Rupert had done this by himself. As if to acknowledge his prowess, he giggled in glee, like a naughty child caught out.

'Rupert!' we chorused, 'What a clever boy!' He bounced up and down on sturdy little legs, milking the moment for all it was worth.

We put him back into kneeling position, hoping for a demonstration, but alas, he struggled and failed. Minutes later we returned to the room to find him standing again. Perseverence had paid off!

Our baby is turning into a little boy!

Your baby

From now on your baby seems continually on the move, in one way or another, so watch out, and be prepared for anything (like attempts to stand up in a slippery bath). He'll also be grasping at all objects within reach so remember to heed the advice about not holding hot liquids while baby's near, and make sure the house is well baby-proofed, with dangerous items out of reach.

Developments to look forward to over the next 6 months

Crawling
Crawling may be achieved any time between now and 12 months. It can start in various ways: often paddling with arms while on the tummy, then inching forward with bottom in the air and legs straight. Some babies, who have not had much time on their tummies, may propel themselves forward on their bottoms instead of crawling.

Standing and cruising
Your baby may pull up to the standing position any time between now and 9 months. The next stage is to cruise around the room supporting himself on the furniture and walls, so protect your pot plants and breakables! But don't get excited and try to rush him into walking independently. It usually takes at least 3 months from pulling up before baby takes his first real steps.

Walking
Walking independently often happens at about 12 months, although it could be just before, or it could be as late as 18 months (and still be classified as normal). Wait until he's been walking in soft shoes for 4 to 5 weeks before investing in his first pair of hard-soled shoes. (You may like to have them cast in bronze when he grows out of them!)

6 MONTHS AND BEYOND

Talking
Suddenly you'll find some of the vocalisation is making sense. A certain sound may be repeated over and over, becoming 'word of the week'. Often the first one is 'dah dah', much to the delight of your partner. Encourage baby by speaking to him often and responding positively when he talks.

Feeding
Soon you'll begin to ease into the routine of 3 to 4 milk feeds a day, and 3 solid meals — which can include yoghurt, ricotta, cottage or grated cheese, egg yolk (scrambled with vegetables, poached or eaten from a finger of toast), fish, minced meat and chicken, rice, pasta, vegetables, fruit, mashed baked beans, soups, mild dhal and sugar-free custard. You'll enjoy baby's earnest attempts to feed himself. It's important to give coarse foods from about 7 months (depending on when you started solids). Most babies will be into finger food by about 8 months (some perhaps as early as 5 or 6 months), and at 12 months they can drink cow's milk, and share in the family meals.

Sleeping
Over the next 6 months, baby will probably be sleeping between 10 and 16 hours a day. This could consist of an overnight sleep of say 10 hours, and morning and afternoon naps of 1 to 2 hours each. If he now rolls onto his tummy to sleep, you need not be unduly concerned.

Teething
Most babies will develop at least several teeth during this period. Some have as many as 8 by the time they reach 12 months while others are still waiting to cut their first.

Toddlerhood
At the end of the year, your baby will have transformed into a little girl or a little boy. Enjoy the closeness and vulnerability of babyhood while you have it. The time passes so fleetingly. Then again, you'll love toddlerhood! The wonderful thing about having children is that it just seems to get better and better.

HELP LINES

Always remember that your child health nurse is the best starting point for any problems. Some family care services are not listed here, because they prefer that you seek referral through your doctor or child health centre.
Note also that some of the 24-hour numbers may often be busy, depending on the time you call and the number of counsellors rostered on. Some will put your call in a queue if the lines are congested, others will take your number via an answering machine and return your call when convenient.

National Help Lines

Australian Multiple Birth Association
02 9875 2404
Referral to state-based volunteers.

Child Support Agency
131 272
For legal support questions.

Lifeline Australia Inc.
24-hour help line 131 114
Offers counselling for all types of crises.

Australian Capital Territory

Canberra One Parent Family Support
06 247 4282
Advice and referrals, home visits, organisation of housing, legal advice, emotional and financial support.

Queen Elizabeth Hospital
24-hour help lines 06 249 7792, 06 248 0813
Specialises in postnatal enquiries (babies to toddlers).

Nursing Mothers' Association of Australia
24-hour help line 06 258 8928

New South Wales

Child Abuse Prevention Service (CAPS)
24-hour help line 02 9716 8000
Freecall 1800 688 009
For parents under stress and general child abuse-related problems.

Child Protection and Family Crisis Service
24-hour crisis line Freecall 1800 066 777
Deals with issues of child protection and child abuse.

Dial-a-Mum
02 9477 6777
8 a.m. to midnight
A confidential listening-ear supplied by trained volunteer mothers.

Family Crisis Service
02 9622 0522
Mon–Fri 6 p.m.–11 p.m., weekends and public holidays 10 a.m.–11 p.m.

Karitane
24-hour help line 02 9794 1852
Freecall 1800 677 961
Residential unit, free day stay services, volunteer home visiting service and specialist service for severe postnatal depression.

Nursing Mothers' Association of Australia
24-hour help line 02 9639 8686

Parent Line
Local call charge from country areas 132055
Mon–Sat 9 a.m.–4.30 p.m.
Counselling service for families with children 0–18 years.

Tresillian Family Care Centres
24-hour help line 02 9569 5400
Freecall 1800 637 357
Residential care, free day stay services and home visits (Outreach).

Northern Territory

Alice Springs Community Services Counsellor
8.30 a.m.–5 p.m. 08 8953 0785
After-hours hotline 1800 188 082

Crisis Line
08 8981 9227
Freecall 1800 019 116
24-hour help line for general counselling. Appointments for personal counselling during business hours can be made at any time. Extensive referral resources for the Northern Territory.

Darwin Family Day Care
08 8945 2945
Referral to services in Katherine, Tenant Creek and other regions of the Northern Territory.

Northern Territory Women's Information Service
Freecall 1800 813 631
Information, advice and referral service.

Nursing Mothers' Association of Australia
24-hour help line 08 8983 2380

Queensland

Children's Community Health Services
07 3862 2333
Freecall 1800 177 279
Advice about parenting.

Family Day Care Association
07 3395 7044
Freecall 1800 177 253
Organises in-home care (at other people's homes) for children of working parents.

Nursing Mothers' Association of Australia
24-hour help line 07 3844 8977

South Australia

Child and Youth Health
08 303 1500
Local call charge from country areas 1300 364 100
Advice for parents with children 0–24 years.

Crisis Care
Local call charge from country areas 13611
After-hours telephone counselling
Mon—Fri 4 p.m.—9 a.m., 24 hours weekends and public holidays

Nursing Mothers' Association of Australia
24-hour help line 08 8339 6783

Parent Support Service
08 374 1809
Flinders Medical Centre 5 p.m.—11 p.m. only

Tasmania

Child Health Association
03 6231 4765
Head office in Hobart offers referral to regional help centres.

Early support for parents
03 6223 2937
Volunteer support for families in their own homes in Hobart.

Lady Gowrie Family Support Service
03 6236 9256
For referrals.

Lady Gowrie Tasmania Resource Service
Freecall 1800 675 416
Offering library service, printed information and videos.

Nursing Mothers' Association of Australia
24-hour help line 03 6223 2609

Parent Information Telephone Assistance Service (PITAS)
Hobart and southern region 03 6233 2700
Launceston and northern region, Walker House 03 6326 6188
Devonport, north-west parent centre 03 6434 6201
State-wide after-hours line for urgent parenting problems 5 p.m.—8 a.m., Freecall 1800 808 178

Victoria

Caroline Chisholm Society
24-hour help line 03 9370 3933
Freecall 1800 134 863
Support for pregnant women and families with children under primary-school age. Qualified staff during the day and volunteers after hours.

Council of Single Mothers and their Children
03 9415 1171
9.30 a.m.—1 p.m.

Crisis Line
24-hour help line 03 9329 0300

Family Life Assistance Group
03 9558 1866

Maternal and Child Health After-hours Service
03 9853 0844
Freecall 1800 134 883
Weekdays 6 p.m. to midnight, weekends and public holidays noon to midnight. For telephone counselling, advice and referral when your local council nurse is not available.

Nursing Mothers' Association of Australia
24-hour help line 03 9878 3304

Women's Information and Referral Service (WIRE)
03 9654 6844
Freecall 1800 136 570
Typing phone for the hearing impaired
03 9654 5124

Western Australia

After-hours Child Health Nurse
09 367 3256
Mon–Fri 5 p.m.–10 p.m., weekends and public holidays 8 a.m.–1 p.m.

Family and Parenting Service
Family Help Line 09 221 2000
Freecall 1800 643 000
Parentline 09 272 1466
Freecall 1800 654 432

Lone Parents' Support Service
09 389 8373
10 a.m.–3.00 p.m.
Advice and referrals for single parents with children 0–16 years.

Ngala Family Resource Centre
09 367 7855
After-hours Child Health Hotline
09 367 3256
Telephone advice, child care, home visits, parent education, day stay and family residential program support for parents with children aged 0–6 years.

Nursing Mothers' Association of Australia
24-hour help line 09 309 5393

Parent Help Centre
Freecall 1800 807 648
Advice, information and counselling from qualified staff.

INDEX

activities, baby 111
activity gym 15, 182, 226
ailments, common 118–19
alcohol and breastfeeding 81–2
amusements, baby 162, 195, 228, 230
   see also games; play
audio cassettes 17, 21

baby
   blues 43–4, 58
   book 17
   caring for 38
   jumper 195
   proofing 213
   safety 16, 213–15, 229, 231
   walker 196
baby-sitting 122
backpack, baby 19, 204–5
bag, baby 13, 72, 191
bassinet 12, 67–8
bath, baby 21
baths, big 167

bathing tips 86–7
bedtime routine 133
bibs 222
   double terry-towelling 8
birth
   after pains 33
   post-caesarean 32–3
   post-vaginal 32
blankets, cellular cotton 12
bleeding, postnatal 22, 33
blues
   baby 43–4, 58
   late afternoon 139
body, your 32–3, 106, 147, 206
books 212, 232
bottle
   carrier, thermal 18
   feeding 18–19, 41–2, 83–6, 164, 197
   warmer, electric 18
bottles, feeding 18
bouncer, baby 15
bras, maternity 23

breastfeeding 28, 39–41, 59, 68, 72,
    76–82, 102–4, 143–5, 158, 165, 183,
    197, 216
  and alcohol 81–2
  difficulties 35–6
  ease 102–3
  feeding on demand 76
  the first breastfeed 34–5
  foods to eat while 81
  foremilk and hindmilk 80–1
  frequency of feeding 36–7
  if you haven't enough milk 103–4
  if your milk doesn't come in 40
  night feeding tips 69
  tips 69, 77–8
  when your milk comes in 39–40
  and working 183
  see also breasts; expressing milk; mastitis;
      nipples; weaning
breasts
  care of 22, 45–7, 78–9
  comfort 164–5
  pads 158
  pump 17, 47–8
  see also nipples
bunny rugs 11–12
burping tips 82

caesarean 32
camera, video 21, 124
capsule, baby 13–14, 58, 225–6
car seat 13–14, 58, 225–6
chair, portable 15
change table 11
checkup, baby's 140–1
child health centre 99–100, 101, 198, 231
childcare 120–1, 142, 185–7, 191
clothes dryer 20
clothing
  postnatal 23
  sizes 8
colic 74, 94

colostrum 35
comforts, cuddly 180–1
communication 212
community resources 101–2
cot 67–8
  from cradle 163
  portable 20
counselling services 189
cradle 12, 67–8
  to cot 163
cradle cap 119
crawling 236
creams 21–2
crying 48–9, 73, 75, 94, 117–18, 120,
    124–5, 137

day-care centres 121
diary, keeping a 118
diet *see* food; meals
dimmer/night light 12
dining out 52–3, 175
discomfort, postnatal 22
dishwasher basket 20
drooling 188
dummies 49–50, 86, 225

entertainment, baby 111, 129, 149–50,
    161–2, 181–2, 192, 195, 228, 230
episiotomy 33–4
exercise 52, 100–1, 146
  see also pelvic floor exercises
expectations versus reality 70–1
expressing milk 17, 48, 142–5
eye contact 123

family care centre 116, 135–6, 148
family day-care 122
fathers 56–9, 89–91, 107, 123–5,
    148–50, 174–5, 191, 207–8, 232–3
feeding
  bibs 8, 220
  equipment, sterilisation of 85–6

INDEX

night 69
patterns 132, 179–80, 237
quantities 164, 216
schedule 70
see also bottle, feeding; breastfeeding; food
first aid 215
food
  adding formula to the diet 216
  basic rules for solids 201–2
  expanding the menu 219
  freezing solids 220
  more on solids 218
  readiness for solids 198
  starting on solids 200–2
foods to eat while breastfeeding 81
formula
  adding to diet 216
  and combining breastfeeding 165, 183, 199, 218–19
  dispenser 18
fun 161–2

games 149–50
  see also activities; amusements; entertainment; play
getting out 98–9, 142, 159, 175
grooming needs 17
growth spurts 146
gymnastic activities 18, 182, 226

hammock, baby 19, 111–12
hands 166
handling techniques 123, 174
hearing 218
help
  home 160
  lines 88, 101, 189, 238–41
highchair 222
holding the baby 38, 58, 123, 155, 174
home
  alone 112

based care 122
help 160
keeping order 194
when first at 54–5, 106
hospital
  rooming-in 31
  routine 30
  telephones 31
  tips 28
  visitors 30–1
housework 63, 194

immunisation 159

jumpers, baby 195
jumpsuits 8

kindergartens 121

legs 166
lifting 38, 58
luxury items 19–21

massage 208
mastitis 79–80, 144, 197, 225
meals, frozen 23, 71, 220
  see also dining out; food
meconium 38
medical kit 16
milestones 24, 60, 92, 108, 126, 152, 176, 192, 210, 234
milk rash 118–19
mobiles 16, 68, 155, 174
mobility 205
monitor, baby 19
moods 161–2
mothers' groups, postnatal 141

nails 38
names 39, 57
nappies 9–10, 50–1, 87–8, 231–2
  wet 38

nappy
  bucket 11
  fasteners 11
  liners 10, 87
  rash 87–8
  wipes 21–2
navels 38
night
  duty 68–9
  feeding 69, 114
  light 12
nighties 9
nipples
  care of 22, 45–7, 78–9
  sore 45
  see also breasts
Nursing Mothers' Association 17, 41, 88, 102

occasional care centres 122
organisation 71–2, 110
overtiredness 73–4

pelvic floor exercises 52, 115, 146
photo album 17
photographs 51, 124
pilchers 10–11
play 129, 181–2, 191
  see also activities; amusements;
    entertainment; games
playgroups 229
posseting 65, 168–71
postnatal depression 188–9
pouch, baby 15, 111
powder 21
power points, safety 16
pram 14
preschools 121, 229–30
proof mat 12–13

reality versus expectations 70–1
reflux 65, 168–71
relaxation tips 98

rest, importance of 63–4, 106, 206
rocking chair 20
routine 70, 105, 113, 114, 118, 132, 133, 156

safety
  baby 213–15, 231
  switches 16
  water-awareness classes 229
school 191, 230
separates 9
settling
  aids 95
  art of 95
  controlled 117–18
  techniques 70, 75, 95–6, 134, 160–1
sex 115, 124
shampoo 21
shoulders, sore 46
shopping
  techniques 123–4
  tips 7–23, 142
showers 167
SIDS see Sudden Infant Death Syndrome
singlets 9
sleeping
  arrangements 65–6
  management 133
  patterns 132, 133, 146, 160–1, 179–80, 237
  position 130
  schedule 70
  through 145, 160–1, 172, 175, 198
  time 96
slings, baby 15, 111
socks 9
solids
  basic rules 201–2
  freezing 220
  more on solids 218
  readiness 198–9
  starting 200–2

INDEX

spontaneity versus routine 156
standing 236
sterilization of feeding equipment 85–6
steriliser, electric steam 18–19
stitches 22
stories 232
stroller 14
Sudden Infant Death Syndrome (SIDS) 32, 66, 13
swaddling 31–2
swing, baby 20, 111–12
switches, safety 16

talking 237
teats 18
teething 202–3, 237
thank-you cards 59
time 138
 to yourself 110–11
Toddler Kindy Gymbaroo 226
toddlerhood 237
tummy time 129–30, 155–6

underblanket, woollen 12–13

video camera 21, 124
visual stimulation 16, 155
vision 68
visitors 112
 controlling 30–1, 56, 105
Vomiting Infants Support Association 170

walkers, baby 196
walking 236
water jug 18
water-awareness classes 229
weaning 224–5
witching hour 106, 208
working
 and breastfeeding 183
women 157–8, 183